THE COMPLETE BOOK OF
DREAMS

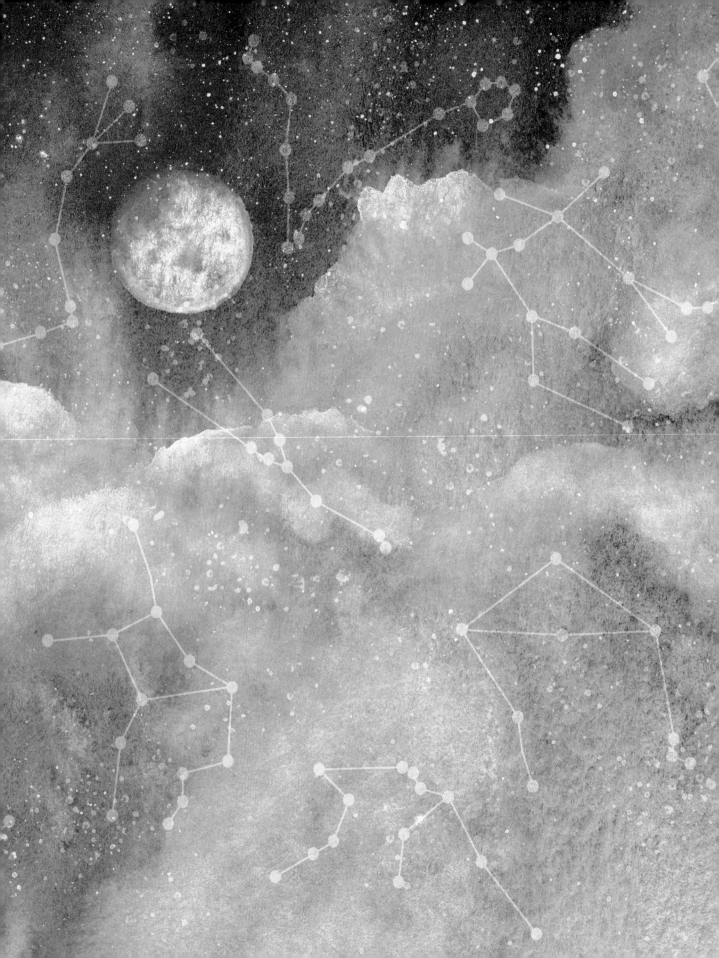

THE COMPLETE BOOK OF
DREAMS

a guide to unlocking the meaning and healing power of your dreams

STEPHANIE GAILING

WELLFLEET

P R E S S

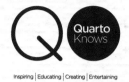

Inspiring | Educating | Creating | Entertaining

Brimming with creative inspiration, how-to projects, and useful information to enrich your everyday life, Quarto Knows is a favorite destination for those pursuing their interests and passions. Visit our site and dig deeper with our books into your area of interest: Quarto Creates, Quarto Cooks, Quarto Homes, Quarto Lives, Quarto Drives, Quarto Explores, Quarto Gifts, or Quarto Kids.

First published in 2020 by Wellfleet Press, an imprint of The Quarto Group
142 West 36th Street, 4th Floor, New York, NY 10018, USA
T (212) 779-4972 F (212) 779-6058 www.QuartoKnows.com

Wellfleet titles are also available at discount for retail, wholesale, promotional, and bulk purchase. For details, contact the Special Sales Manager by email at specialsales@quarto.com or by mail at The Quarto Group, Attn: Special Sales Manager, 100 Cummings Center Suite 265D, Beverly, MA 01915 USA.

10 9 8 7 6 5 4 3 2 1

ISBN: 978-1-57715-213-2

Library of Congress Control Number: 2020939639

Publisher: Rage Kindelsperger | Creative Director: Laura Drew | Managing Editor: Cara Donaldson
Senior Editor: John Foster | Cover Design: Sosha Davis | Interior Design: Kate Smith |
Illustrations by Sosha Davis with the exception of pages 36, 80, 89, 92, 142, 162, and 213 © Shutterstock

Printed in China

This book provides general information on various widely known and widely accepted theories on sleep and dream interpretation. However, it should not be relied upon as recommending or promoting any specific diagnosis or method of treatment for a particular condition, and it is not intended as a substitute for medical advice or for direct diagnosis and treatment of a medical condition by a qualified physician. Readers who have questions about a particular condition, possible treatments for that condition, or possible reactions from the condition or its treatment should consult a physician or other qualified health-care professional.

CONTENTS

introduction

What did you dream last night? It may have been illuminating or confounding, captivating or relatively uninspiring. Perhaps it was a joyous adventure like none other, or a scene so upsetting it rattled you to the core. It may have included people, places, and events that were all too familiar, or those that were seemingly bizarre and unrecognizable. Likely, it defied your ordinary perception of how space and time operate, leaving you wondering just from where this symphony of mesmerizing visions emerged. Assuming, that is, if you remembered your dreams. On par with the mystery that surrounds what they mean and where they come from is the question of where they go and why they seem to dissolve so quickly. Owing to their evanescent quality, some people even believe that they don't have them at all. However, we all dream.

It is one of the things that unites us, an activity common to all of humanity. What also unites us is our shared interest in dreams, this enigmatic subject that has intrigued people throughout history. For as much as dreams are a phenomenon that occurs when we sleep, they are not necessarily cordoned off from our waking experiences. People have continually looked to their dreams for insights on how to navigate the opportunities and challenges that comprise their daily lives. We only need to look to language to observe this interplay. In addition to signifying "a series of thoughts, images, or emotions occurring during sleep," the *Merriam-Webster* dictionary notes that the word *dream* also has numerous other meanings. We use it when we want to signify "something notable for its beauty, excellence, or enjoyable quality," or "a strongly desired goal or purpose," or even "something that fully satisfies a wish." As such, as mystical and enigmatic as our nighttime dreams are, there's a perception that they are somehow akin to our daytime visions, aims, and desires. Before we explore how to tap into the benefits that our dreams can offer us, let's gain a historical perspective that will allow us to see how they were viewed throughout time. Doing so is not only fascinating, but provides us with access to a spectrum of understanding as we quest to know more about what dreams are and what they mean.

Ancient Dream Wisdom

Since antiquity, dreams have maintained a very important role in cultures across the globe, extolled for their visionary wisdom. In fact, as far back as the ancient Sumerian civilization, dreams served as guides for important decision making. For example, in clay relics dating from about 2125 BCE, we find cuneiform inscriptions recounting dreams experienced by Gudea, the ruler of the Mesopotamian city-state of Lagash. In these prophetic oneiric visions, the king received not only encouragement to build E-ninnu, a revered temple dedicated to the god Ninĝirsu, but also design details that he then used to construct the sacred site.

Another famous dream series that dates to this historical period is of those featured in *The Epic of Gilgamesh*. Prized as the oldest extant piece of literature, the tale includes numerous action-guiding dreams had by the Mesopotamian king Gilgamesh. It is inscribed on clay tablets in the Library of Ashurbanipal, dating from the seventh century BCE, which also feature other carvings detailing the interpretation of numerous dream symbols. Of course, when we look to ancient wisdom, we often turn toward the Egyptians, who themselves held a high regard for dreams. A prized example of oneiric literature is the *Ramesside Dream Manual*, found in the famed

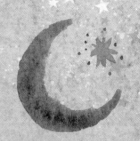

The Oneiric Language of Dreams

As you read this book, you'll come across words like *oneiric* and *oneirology*. The former signifies something that pertains to dreams or dreaming, and the latter, the scientific study of dreams. These words derive from the Greek *oneiros*, which means "to dream"; in Greek mythology, the gods of dreams — including Hypnos, Phobetor, and Phantasos — were collectively referred to as the Oneiroi. Dream interpreters were classically known as oneirocritics, with one of the most famous ancient dream books, dating from the second century CE, entitled *Oneirocritica*.

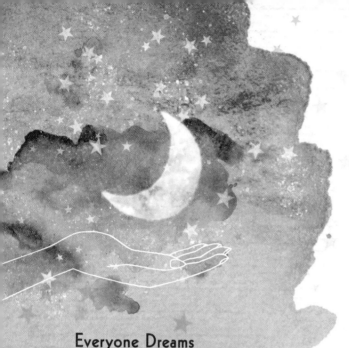

Everyone Dreams

How often have you heard someone say that they don't dream? Perhaps you've said this as well, considering yourself a person who never experiences the nighttime reverie of oneiric visions. Well, as it turns out, it's thought that everyone dreams; it's just that some people don't remember having them when they awaken. So, don't worry — with intention and practice (including some of the tips featured in chapter 12), you, too, can have a dream life.

Chester Beatty Papyri (c. 1250–1100 BCE). It contains more than one hundred dreams, their explanations, and a qualifier as to whether the dream is considered to be a "good" or "bad" one.

As the ancient Greek and Roman civilizations flourished, so did the perception of another benefit that dreams held: that of their role in medicine and healing. Not only did esteemed physicians and philosophers of the time — including Hippocrates, Aristotle, and Galen — promote theories on how dreams were intertwined with health, but hundreds of dream sanctuaries were established across the region for those seeking cures. Called Asklepieia, these sacred temples are perhaps the best-known examples of venues where dream incubation — ritualized sleep undertaken in a holy site — was performed. Dream incubation dates back to earlier Babylonian times and was practiced by cultures throughout the world; for instance, there are mentions that in ancient Japan, supplicants would sleep in Buddhist and Shinto temples in hopes of receiving a healing dream.

Religions the world over have also acknowledged the mystery and power of dreams, detailed in many doctrinal texts. This includes both the Old and New Testaments, in which there are twenty-one references to dreams. One of the most cited is the story of Joseph and Pharaoh that appears in Genesis. In it, Joseph successfully interprets Pharaoh's two dreams, noting that they are actually reflections of one message that augured seven years of plenty, followed by seven years of famine. In the Book of Daniel, we also learn of the story of Daniel, who interpreted a visionary dream of King Nebuchadnezzar. In each of these stories, it's emphasized that both Joseph and Daniel were not the source of the dream interpretations, but rather messengers of those that came from a divine source.

There are several mentions of dreams in the Qur'an. These include reference to ones had by the prophet Muhammad, as well as the retelling of the dreams of Joseph and Abraham cited in the Old Testament. In the Islamic tradition, it's generally thought that there are three types of dreams one can have: ones that are true and divinely inspired; those that arise from within oneself, reflecting one's psychological state; and bad dreams that arise from evil spirits.

Dreaming Throughout the Centuries

Interest in dreams continued throughout the Middle Ages. In medieval Europe, most people believed that, in addition to some

The Dreams of Daniel's Artistic Influence

The *Somniale Danielis*, also referred to as *The Dreams of Daniel*, had a powerful impact upon numerous dreamers during the Middle Ages and beyond, including some quite famous ones. It was thought to have influenced how Dante Alighieri wove dreams through *The Divine Comedy*, as well as the way in which the Italian poet Giovanni Boccaccio addressed them in his works, including *Amorosa Visione* and *The Decameron*. And Leonardo Da Vinci is said to have owned a copy of the *Somniale Danielis*, which he used to interpret his own dreams. One can only imagine how his oneiric visions informed his artistic and technical works, notably in light of Da Vinci's reflection that "the eye sees a thing more clearly in dreams than the imagination awake."

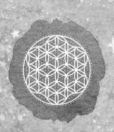

The Gates of Horn and Ivory

Dreams were accorded prophetic potential throughout history. However, that doesn't mean that people believed all oneiric visions foretold the future. Often referred to as "true" and "false" dreams, they also were sometimes alluded to as those that came through the gates of horn (those that held veracity) and those that came through the gates of ivory (those that were false or misleading). The reference for this comes from Homer in *The Odyssey*, when he writes of Penelope speaking with an incognito Odysseus about a dream she had about his return, noting that not every dream is one that offers prescient insights.

dreams being divinely inspired, others could arise from mental stress or physiological origins. Some dreams were seen to have oracular properties, while others contained telltale signs that revealed future events. People viewed certain dreams to offer clear and obvious directionality, while others were veiled and required the assistance of a dream interpreter, or dream guidebook, to understand. Consequently, dream guides began to flourish during these times. Among these were the A to Z dream dictionaries, similar to the ones that are still popular today. Coming into fashion in the ninth century CE, among the most notable of these oneiric glossaries is the *Somniale Danielis (The Dreams of Daniel)*, dedicated to the prophet from the Old Testament.

With dreams seen as having the potential for prophecy, a question that has coursed itself throughout history is whether or not an oneiric vision had veracity or would manifest. To assess this in the Middle Ages, people would often turn to books known as dream lunaries. After having a dream, you'd look up the date in this book, which would tell you the current phase of the Moon: depending upon what it was, the book would note whether your dream was likely to come true or not. In the twelfth century, two other types of oneiric books became popular. Among them were treatises that addressed and interpreted themes that would arise in dreams, such as the famed *Oneirocritica* by Artemidorus, originally written in the second century, and Pascalis Romanus's twelfth-century *Liber Thesauri Occulti*. The latter included insights into how oneiric visions can provide diagnostic and therapeutic health insights. Also popular at this time were guides known as mantic alphabets; while these didn't actually provide insights into the dreams themselves, people would consult them after awakening from an oneiric-filled sleep to gain general predictions for the future. All of these dream books maintained popularity until around the seventeenth century, when they began falling out of fashion. Some posit that this was the effect of the Catholic Church censoring and denouncing dream texts. While it had earlier put forth its own dream theory, fusing Christian and Pagan tenets, the Church may have been unsupportive of people directly connecting to their dreams because it harnessed a sense of individual spiritual agency.

The poetry of the nineteenth-century Romantic period is studded with examples of dream poems, those that would recount oneiric journeys, or those that used dreams as a story-telling instrument. This was a time in which individual thought and personal feelings emerged from the shadows and was highlighted in art; many suggest that some of this period's poetic works presaged the notion of the unconscious, which those in the field of psychology later made popular. Within Romanticism, we find an example of one of the most oneirically inspired works of modern times: Samuel Taylor Coleridge's *Kubla Khan* (also called *A Vision in a Dream*). Soon after, the idea that dreams had an oracular function and offered the ability to glimpse into the future again become a popular premise. In the mid- to late-nineteenth century, we see books combining dream interpretation with other mantic systems similar to the books of medieval Europe. Two of the more popular books of this genre included Madam Le Marchand's *Fortune Teller and Dream Dictionary* and Napoleon's *Oraculum and Dream Book*.

Through the Lens of Psyche

As we have seen throughout history, many people believed that dreams gave insights into the present and could foretell the future. The past wasn't really something considered when it came to the realm of dreams. That is, until the early twentieth century. That's when psychology began making inroads into popular culture, and an Austrian psychotherapist named Sigmund Freud catalyzed the idea that dream content stemmed from issues from one's childhood. Additionally, the emphasis on dreams coming from an external divine source made room for the idea that they originated from within, from the depths of the unconscious mind. Dreams began to be further seen as providing prized insights into one's psychological orientation and emotional nature, something for which they continue to be heralded today. To forge an understanding as to how dreams play a role in psychological well-being, let's look at the perspectives held by two pioneers recognized to have played a pivotal role in shaping modern dream theory — Sigmund Freud and Carl Jung — as well as several others who made great contributions to the field.

SIGMUND FREUD (1856 – 1939)

With the 1899 publishing of Sigmund Freud's seminal work *The Interpretation of Dreams*, a new chapter was ushered in related to the attention given to dreams, both by laypersons and those in the medical community. Referred to as the father of psychoanalysis, Freud thought dreams played an essential role in understanding a person's hidden impulses, as well as their repressed sexual wishes. Freud is famous for calling them "the royal road to the unconscious." He asserted that the dream that is remembered (the manifest dream) is but a disguised version

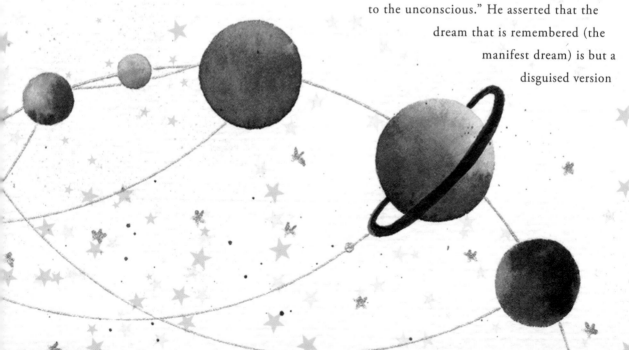

of what it really signified (the latent dream). He viewed techniques such as free association instrumental in helping patients access the latter. In addition to assisting the dreamer discharge the energy of forbidden wishes within their psyche, Freud perceived the disguised dream as playing the role of the guardian of sleep: he believed that without its obfuscation, a dream would be so upsetting that it could keep a person from getting a good night's rest. Since Freud, many psychologists have put forth numerous other dream theories, the constructions of which oftentimes were built upon or refuted those he proposed.

CARL JUNG (1875 – 1961)

Another vanguard in the field was the Swiss psychoanalyst Carl Jung, the founder of analytical psychology. Jung was a disciple of Freud's until their now-famous split, which was caused by their different perspectives on the role of the unconscious that mirrored their differing views on dreams. Instead of seeing dreams as signals of disturbance, Jung saw them as outlets of creative expression. He felt that dreams were pivotal for obtaining an aim he viewed as utterly important: that of attaining individuation, the embrace of the wholeness of self and one's unique destiny. He was a strong proponent of the wisdom that messages from the unconscious

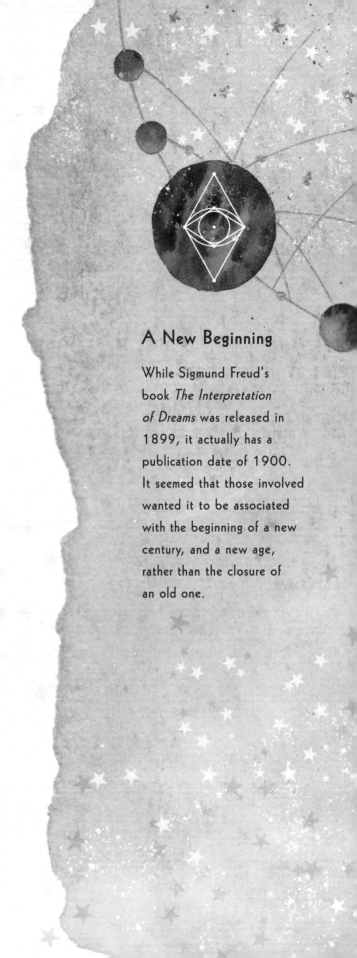

A New Beginning

While Sigmund Freud's book *The Interpretation of Dreams* was released in 1899, it actually has a publication date of 1900. It seemed that those involved wanted it to be associated with the beginning of a new century, and a new age, rather than the closure of an old one.

brought forth in dreams. Jung pioneered the dreamwork technique known as Active Imagination. He also emphasized that while dream images were personal to the dreamer, many were derived from universal mythic symbols (which he called archetypes). From this perspective, he felt that dreams could serve as a lens into the collective unconscious, denoted to be an understanding that is shared by all of humanity.

ALFRED ADLER (1870 – 1937)

Alfred Alder saw dreams as "dress rehearsals for life." He felt that they were practical in their purpose, offering a person insight into how they could solve problems and navigate through situations that they may face in the future. He saw them as mirroring motivations and aspirations intrinsic to the dreamer, and that in them we sometimes exhibit behaviors that compensate for the weaknesses we perceive ourselves to have.

FRITZ PERLS (1893 – 1970)

According to Fritz Perls, the founder of gestalt therapy, every image and character in the dream represents an aspect of the dreamer. He posited that their inclusion in the dream allows for a recognition and subsequent reintegration of rejected or disowned parts of ourselves. Using his approach, a person reenacts their dream through taking on the perspective of each element that was featured in it, giving voice to what it has to share.

ERICH FROMM (1900 – 1980)

Erich Fromm eschewed some of the central dream theory tenets held by both Freud and Jung, while also mirroring others. Author of *The Forgotten Language*, he noted that dreams reflected both biological drives and wisdom that goes beyond our waking thoughts. He posited that dreams were a symbolic language that was common to everyone, one that could be accessed when we slept and unencumbered by the waking-life constraints of social conditioning.

JAMES HILLMAN (1926 – 2011)

James Hillman, the founder of archetypal psychology and author of *The Dream and the Underworld*, advocated that the virtue inherent in a dream resides within the images themselves. Rather than analyzing them and seeing how they coordinated with a person's waking life, he urged people to "stick with the image." To do so, he suggested describing the image and asking questions of it, rather than interpreting it, allowing the image to naturally unfold and reveal its essential nature.

The Sway of Science

A new chapter in the history books of dreams began in 1953, when Eugene Aserinksy and Nathaniel Kleitman published a research paper in the journal *Science* noting their discovery of rapid eye movement (REM) sleep. During this period of slumber, not only do the eyes move in tandem at a quicker pace than in other sleep phases, but the brain is activated in a somewhat similar manner as when we are awake. The publication of their research laid the foundation for subsequent explorations in dreaming, given that it established a physiological correlate for its occurrence.

One of the outcomes of their discovery was the emergence of theories — including those postulated by leaders in the field of psychiatry — that dreams are not solely the result of our psyches offering revelatory insights about who we are. Take sleep researcher and Harvard faculty member J. Alan Hobson, MD, for example. He, along with his colleague Robert McCarley, proposed the now-famous activation-synthesis hypothesis. This neurobiological theory suggests that it's actually neurophysiological processes, not psychological stirrings, that are the prime factors responsible for the imagery and characteristics inherent in dreams.

Another luminary who proposed a physiological function for REM sleep was Francis Crick, of DNA helix-discovery fame. In the 1980s, he and his colleague Graeme Mitchison advanced the reverse learning theory that asserts that the function of dream sleep is to clear the brain of unnecessary neural connections that impede upon memory. From this perspective, instead of

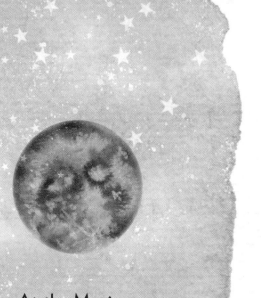

At the Movies

Movies sometimes feel like waking dreams, as we get to leave our daily world behind and climb into the imaginative world offered by the film. That said, there are some films in which dreams actually play a starring role, including *Total Recall*, *Inception*, *Waking Life*, and *Dreams*, the last one a movie based upon the director Akira Kurosawa's own oneiric journeys.

being an experience in which the unconscious mind reveals valuable hidden insights, they submit that REM dreaming discards what's considered insignificant and without value.

The perspectives that have been derived from oneirology have added to the ongoing multi-versed inquiry into understanding the phenomenon of dreams. And yet, regardless of these biologically based theories, most people still believe that oneiric visions provide us with a wealth of access into the depths of personal awareness. That dreams are a stage upon which striking insights come forth supports the belief that they are also a source of breakthrough ideas. As we're about to see, this impact is not only limited to our personal lives, but extends to the collective as well.

A Canvas of Creativity

As you likely know from your own dreams, they are a robust canvas of the imaginative. It's therefore not surprising that the Land of Nod and the landscape of both art and invention form a beautiful kinship, especially with authors, musicians, and artists. There have been numerous accounts of authors giving credit to their dreams for some of their greatest opuses. For example, Mary Shelley noted that it was in a dream that she had a vision that forged the basis of the idea for her famous novel *Frankenstein*. E.B. White has shared that the character of Stuart Little appeared to him in a dream. Stephen King has said that he received some of the fundamental ideas for a book that would later become *Misery* in a dream he had while on an airplane. Another famous writer who found their dreams to be a reservoir of creativity is Robert Louis Stevenson. The novelist recounted in his duly named essay "A Chapter on Dreams" that he discovered the idea for the famous window scene in *The Strange Case of Dr. Jekyll and Mr. Hyde* in a dream. This dream didn't appear out of the blue, though; rather, it occurred after days in which he spent a multitude of waking hours trying to figure out ways to navigate a creative impasse. As we'll see in chapter 11, daytime rumination on a challenge often catalyzes our ability to experience a breakthrough in our nighttime dreams.

In addition to authors, numerous musicians — Paul McCartney, Jimi Hendrix, Michael Stipe, and others — have also remarked that it was in their dreams that the seeds for songs emerged. And, as it turns out, these weren't just any old songs, but legendary ones, such as "Yesterday," "Purple Haze," and "It's the End of the World as We Know It (And I Feel Fine)," respectively. Likewise, the canvas of dreams also served as inspiration for the canvas of artists. American painter and printmaker Jasper Johns has said that the idea for his iconic *Flags* painting came to him in a dream. And as we'll see on page 83, Salvador Dalí created a system wherein he could preserve the hallucinogenic-like visions from his hypnagogic dreams and use them for his paintings.

A Laboratory for Invention

In addition to being a source of some amazing artwork, dreams have been cited as the laboratory that brought forth some truly revolutionary inventions. Among his other accomplishments, organic chemist August Kekulé is known for deciphering the compositional structure of the benzene molecule. He had shared that its circular organization came to him in a daytime dream in which he envisioned an uberous-like image of a snake swallowing its own tail.

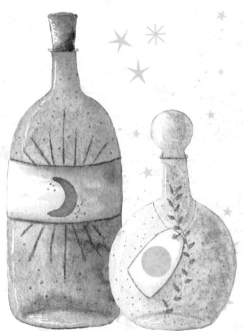

Native Traditions

In traditional cultures, the separation between conscious states is not as demarcated as many portend, and the waking mind isn't granted such hierarchical importance that it supersedes the value of the realities that one experiences while dreaming. In many Native American cultures, wisdom from the spirits and the ancestors is thought to come through dreams, and shamans help tribal members to understand what theirs mean. In many African cultures, dreaming plays an important role in society, as well as in their approach to healing. It's also said that the Maori of New Zealand believe that when a person sleeps, their spirit can leave the body, and that dreams are the mirror of what they experience. In addition to interpreting the content of their dreams, they look to body movements made during sleep; known collectively as *takiri*, some are thought to be auspicious and others not.

Another important breakthrough in chemistry was also accorded to a dream. While writing *Principles of Chemistry*, Dmitri Mendeleev was trying to figure out a system to organize the chemical elements. After struggling with it for three days, he spontaneously had a dream in which an innovative design appeared, what has come to be known as the Periodic Table of Elements.

Chemistry isn't the only province for problem-solving dreams. Medicine, and specifically Nobel-Prize-winning medical discoveries, is another one. In 1923, surgeon Frederick Banting and a colleague were awarded the esteemed prize for the discovery of insulin; as it were, the idea for the experiment that led to its discovery came to Banting in a dream he had one evening. Another dream that led to the winning of a Nobel Prize was had by pharmacologist Otto Lewi, who discovered that nerve conduction was the result of chemical interplay rather than electrical signaling. The inspiration for his finding appeared to him in quite a persistent vision. After having a dream that demonstrated the details of an experiment to undertake, he woke up and wrote it down. However, when looking at it later, he realized he couldn't make out his scribbled notes. As it turns out, the next evening he had the very same dream, which he remembered and whose ideas he subsequently, and successfully, put into motion. In an ironic twist, it turns out that another of the actions of the neurotransmitter he discovered, acetylcholine, increases during REM sleep, the period in which we are thought to have the most vivid of dreams.

Dreams have also spurred the invention of everyday objects. Elias Howe credited one for helping him figure out the design of the sewing machine. And Larry Page, the co-founder of Google, often shares that it was in a dream that the idea for the search engine came to him. Noting this, his suggestion "When a really great dream shows up, grab it" seems like valuable advice.

Dreaming Today

In the last few years, there's been a sleep revolution, which not only served as the title of Arianna Huffington's best-selling book, *The Sleep Revolution*, on the subject, but has also inspired multitudes of people to become more interested in the importance of slumber, and how to get more of it. Concurrently, more and more people are turning toward their dreams, curious as to the power that they hold. And with that, dreams continue to break out of the confines of the counseling room. They're serving as the subject of countless conversations, the focus of numerous online articles, a topic for an array of books, and a realm for dedicated medical research. And if you're tech-inclined, you can explore both your own dreams as well as those of others across the globe through an array of websites and phone apps. As people today continue to pursue a life of greater well-being, including gaining the expanded awareness necessary to navigate these complex times, there's a growing interest in the numinous, as well as approaches that elevate conscious empowerment. Dreams fit this bill beautifully.

As we've seen, dreams gift us with a wide range of rewards. They can shine a light into the inner recesses of our mind so that we can further understand oft-shrouded desires, motivations, and potentials. They offer us insights that can augment our holistic health. They can be powerful tools for enhancing creativity and amplifying our problem-solving abilities, while also helping us tap into a broader universal understanding.

How to Use This Book

I have written *The Complete Book of Dreams* to help you access these rewards and elevate your well-being. I hope that this book inspires your connection to your dream life so that you can live the life of which you've always dreamed. As you will discover, it is both a reference and a guidebook. In it, you'll find troves of information that will further forge your understanding of and appreciation for the power of dreams. Plus, the book includes a wealth of simple exercises and other practical how-tos designed to take your dreaming to the next level. It is organized into four parts:

Part I: Sleep
Since to dream well you need to sleep well, in this part of the book you'll learn about the importance of slumber and natural ways to get more of it.

Part II: Dreams
These chapters feature an exploration of the dreaming mind and a survey of the wide range of dreams that we may have.

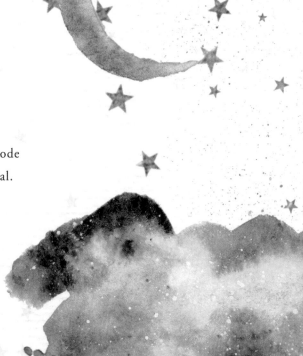

Part III: Dreamwork Practices
In this section, you'll learn an array of strategies to remember your dreams, as well as document and decode them so that you can tap into their powerful potential.

Part IV: Inspiring Children's Dreams
The final two chapters provide you with ways to customize the book's insights for children so that you can inspire their sleep and dreams.

The Complete Book of Dreams can be read in numerous ways. One approach is to read it cover to cover, moving through it as it progresses from insights on sleep to an exploration of dreams. Or, you can dive right into any chapter without having to read another; so, for example, if you're interested in amplifying your dream recall, or accessing strategies to sleep better, or seeing how astrology and dreams sync together, or any number of distinct topics featured in this book, you can go straight to that chapter and learn more about that realm. Whether you read the book sequentially or one chapter at a time, you'll see that there are many cross-references included throughout which point you to ancillary information featured in another area; therefore, flowing between different parts is a third way you may find yourself reading *The Complete Book of Dreams*.

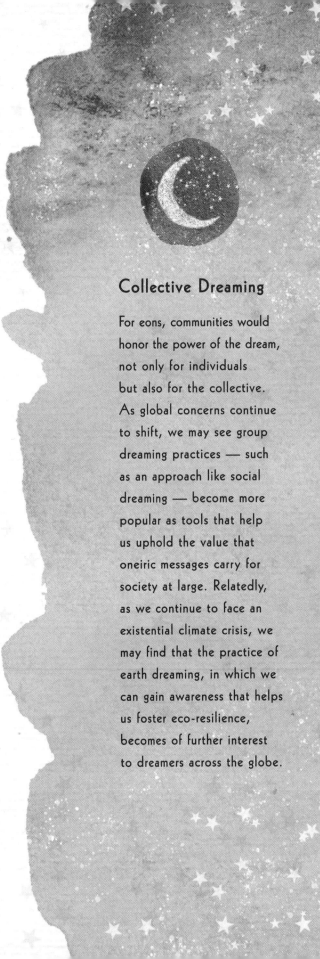

Collective Dreaming

For eons, communities would honor the power of the dream, not only for individuals but also for the collective. As global concerns continue to shift, we may see group dreaming practices — such as an approach like social dreaming — become more popular as tools that help us uphold the value that oneiric messages carry for society at large. Relatedly, as we continue to face an existential climate crisis, we may find that the practice of earth dreaming, in which we can gain awareness that helps us foster eco-resilience, becomes of further interest to dreamers across the globe.

PART 1:

sleep

CHAPTER ONE

EXPLORING SLEEP

Before we enter the world of dreams, let's explore the realm of sleep. After all, we need to sleep well to dream well. And, of course, we need to sleep well because it helps to keep us well. Not only are we filled with more energy and clarity when we're well rested, but a continuing stream of research supports that getting adequate sleep is integral to optimal health and well-being.

It would seem that sleep — as natural as it is — is something that we would naturally have an amiable relationship with, something that would be effortlessly woven into our lives. But, unfortunately, as many of us know, that's far from true. In our modern-day lives, we wrestle with sleep, with our slumber struggles running the gamut. Some people don't prioritize it, laboring to find the interest — let alone the time — to carve out the hours necessary to feel well rested. Consider the often-cited phrase "I'll sleep when I'm dead." With many claiming this as their rallying cry, it reflects how our society's heightened valuation on productivity and achievement often usurps the value we place upon getting a good night's rest. And then there are other people who enjoy sleep and want nothing more than to have it be a trusted and reliable part of their lives. Yet, for one reason or another, they find themselves in the throes of obstacles that keep them from consistent lengthy sojourns to the Land of Nod. That the global sleep-aid industry was valued at almost $70 billion in 2017, and set to grow to almost $102 billion by 2023, is a testament to the collective challenge we face. So is the 2016 finding by the U.S. Centers for Disease Control and Prevention that over one-third of the nation's adults don't get the recommended hours of sleep each night.

Wherever you are on this spectrum, whether you're a sleep admirer or avoider, this chapter and the following three are for you. You'll learn just why sleep is at the bedrock of well-being, how to embrace it, natural approaches that will help you get more of it, and ways to design your bedroom to transform it into a sleep and dream sanctuary. However, before we dive into all of that, let's start with an even more fundamental question: Just what is this thing we call sleep and why is it so important?

What Is Sleep?

Sleep is ubiquitous. Humans sleep. Animals sleep. Even bacteria and some plants exhibit behavior that approximates sleep, in sync with a rhythm that's connected to light and dark. But it's quite a mystery, this thing called sleep, one that's intrigued and puzzled philosophers, physicians, and scientists throughout history.

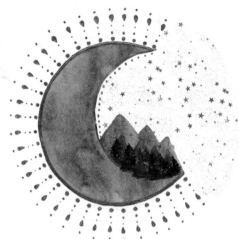

Of course, there are some things we do know about it. We know that it's a biological necessity. Not only because of how we feel when we don't do it, but also because it's an actual must: in a battle between wakefulness and sleep, when we've gone past a certain amount of time being awake, sleep will always be crowned champion. We also know that sleep is quite different than wakefulness. During slumber, we must maintain a prone position and have our eyes closed. We're also unable to move as we do during the day. Our physiological functioning, for the most part, is downshifted as we rest, with vital repair functions occurring. However, this thing we call sleep is not one continuous, undifferentiated activity. As you'll see in chapter 5, sleep has an architecture that is characterized by numerous different stages, each with its own hallmark characteristic (including how dreams are expressed). And while we may assume that sleep is all rest and repose, it is not necessarily a time of complete brain inactivity. As we'll continue to explore, during REM sleep — the period in which it's thought that the most vivid dreams occur — our brain activity is energized in a somewhat similar way as it is when we're awake.

WHY DO WE SLEEP?

Although everyone agrees that sleep is compulsory, there's still no full consensus on just why this is, what occurs during slumber that makes it a prerequisite for life. Here are some of the theories that have been proposed along the way. It seems that none of them completely provides a thorough explanation, and yet, each one does give us a periscope into some of the vital functions that sleep offers. Given the concentrated focus afforded to the arena of sleep, it isn't surprising if new postulates, perhaps ones that even weave in some of these existing theories, continue to be put forward.

Inactivity Theory

The thought: The stillness and quiet that is inherent in sleeping is a survival mechanism, as it keeps animals out of harm's way at night. Modern sleep is an adaptation of this.

Energy Conservation Theory

The thought: Our metabolism slows down during sleep, reducing energy requirements and allowing us to recharge and replenish energy stores.

Restorative Theory

The thought: Important body functions occur mostly or solely during sleep. These include tissue repair, muscle growth, protein synthesis, cell division, and the release of growth hormone.

Neuroplasticity Theory

The thought: A more recent theory that proposes that sleep allows for brain development through the formation of new neural connections, compensating for

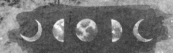

An Ancient Perspective on Why We Sleep

Deciphering what causes us to sleep has captivated people for quite some time. In fact, it significantly predates our modern-day axioms, with one of the first documented theories of sleep posited by Alcmaeon of Croton in the fifth century BCE. This visionary medical theorist hypothesized that sleep was connected to the shifting patterns of blood flow. When the blood withdraws from the body's surface to the larger veins within, sleep occurs, and when it returns to the surface, we awaken. And while we may now find this explanation a bit rudimentary, that it so early on forged a basis of further study — which influenced other notable scholars including Hippocrates — is quite a testament to our ongoing collective intrigue with this mystery called sleep.

injuries and aiding in memory consolidation. Additionally, beneficial brain structural changes occur while we sleep, including the expansion of space between cells, which allows for wastes such as beta-amyloid (the accumulation of which is associated with Alzheimer's disease) to be flushed away.

The Health Benefits of Sleep

While scientists may be equivocal about the overarching mechanisms of why we sleep, research has unequivocally found significant health benefits of doing so. Scientific studies have shown that getting sufficient sleep leads to a longer life. The following findings regarding the health-promoting benefits of sleep may help us understand why.

HEALTHY BODY WEIGHT

Insufficient sleep — consistently getting an average of less than 6 hours each night — is associated with an increased risk of obesity. One proposed reason for this is that skimping on sleep is linked to hormonal changes associated with weight gain. Those who sleep less have been found to have increased levels of ghrelin, a hormone that increases appetite. They have also been found to have reduced levels of leptin, a biochemical messenger that contributes to the feeling of satiety and helps regulate energy expenditure.

HEART HEALTH

Getting inadequate sleep has been associated with a greater risk of having high blood pressure and coronary artery disease. The underlying reasons for this extend beyond both elevated body weight and increased blood sugar levels both negatively impacting cardiovascular health. It may also be related to the finding that short sleep is correlated with higher levels of inflammatory markers and stress hormones.

IMMUNE HEALTH

One outcome of the lack of sleep is the concomitant reduction in immune-supportive molecules known as cytokines. Those deficient in sleep have been found to be more apt to get sick after being exposed to a virus. One of the associative factors for this connection may be simple: when we're exhausted, we're more likely to be stressed, initiating a cascade of body chemicals that dampen our immune response.

BLOOD SUGAR BALANCE

Insufficient sleep may disturb the mechanisms that keep our blood glucose levels within a certain range. Sleep plays an essential, although not yet fully elucidated, role in blood sugar regulation, with sleep deprivation linked to insulin resistance and lowered glucose tolerance.

BETTER MEMORY AND LEARNING

Memory consolidation occurs during sleep, with items shuttled from short-term to long-term memory. Additionally, reduced sleep has also been associated with a compromised ability to concentrate. And, with one of the functions of sleep being the cleaning out of toxins, such as beta-amyloid, poor sleep may enhance our risk of health conditions such as Alzheimer's disease.

EMOTIONAL HEALTH

Lack of sleep may cause alterations in both brain chemistry and hormonal homeostasis, which can lead to depression and anxiety.

The Collective Toll of Inadequate Sleep

In addition to how it impacts our individual health, sleep deprivation bears a significant collective cost. After all, it impacts productivity and alertness, and can cause accidents. Being awake for 17 to 19 hours translates to performing at a similar capacity as those who have a blood alcohol level content of 0.05 percent (in the U.S., 0.08 percent is the threshold to be considered driving under the influence). As it turns out, drowsy driving is the leading cause of crashes and highway fatalities. And when it comes to the workplace, the consequences can be seen there as well: those who are sleep-deprived have about a 150 percent higher risk of being injured on the job. It thus may not surprise you that some of the most devastating accidents in recent history — including the *Challenger* explosion, the Exxon Valdez oil spill, and the Chernobyl nuclear plant meltdown — are thought to have been caused by workers who were sleep-deprived.

Research has linked lack of sleep to higher circulating levels of the stress hormone cortisol. And it may not just be your subjective observation that you get along better with your partner when you're well rested: studies have shown that having adequate sleep may lead to greater satisfaction within relationships.

What Is Adequate Sleep?

The amount of sleep we need depends upon our age, life stage, and health status. And it also depends upon whom you ask, with different organizations in different countries — and even those within the same nation — having their own guidelines. Since the daily target goals are relatively similar, to get a general picture, let's look at those offered by the National Sleep Foundation (NSF). Remember that these recommendations are for the average person. Owing to their innate nature, some people are short sleepers (requiring fewer hours) and some long sleepers (requiring more hours), needing a different amount to maintain their vitality.

Life Stage	*Recommended Daily Sleep*
Newborns (0–3 months)	14–17 hours
Infants (4–11 months)	12–15 hours
Toddlers (1–2 years)	11–14 hours
Preschoolers (3–5 years)	10–13 hours
Children (6–13 years)	9–11 hours
Teenagers (14–17 years)	8–10 hours
Younger adults (18–25 years)	7–9 hours
Adults (26–64 years)	7–9 hours
Older adults (65+years)	7–8 hours

BARRIERS TO SLEEPING WELL

There are numerous reasons that people may not get adequate sleep. For many, there's a feeling that there's just not enough time in the day. Economic pressures have people working longer hours while also maintaining childcare responsibilities that were traditionally assumed by community members. A desire to "stay connected," as well as carve out time to unwind, has the average person spending close to 5 hours a day engaged in social media, messaging platforms, and television watching. With awake time seeming limited, we may eat into our sleep time to find the hours to do all we feel we need to get done.

There are other factors as well, some that are biological in nature. Whether it's a natural process, like menopause or aging, or a health disorder, like restless leg syndrome or untreated obstructive sleep apnea, there are physiological reasons that may underlie an inability to get a restful night's sleep. And let us not forget the stress and worry that rile us up at different points in our lives and keep us tossing and turning.

Some also assert that one of our most hailed technologies is also a key perpetrator in our losing battle to get adequate rest. As it turns out, the nineteenth-century introduction of artificial light shifted our relationship to sleep. It, along with other advances, played a role in catalyzing the Industrial Revolution, which reframed the concept of productivity and workers' schedules — including their natural sleep/wake cycles. Additionally,

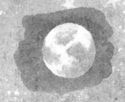

Sleep's Poetic License

Like everything that captivates us in life, sleep has been a province for poets. Through their artistry, we can awaken even further to the dynamic place that it holds for us in our lives. Here are some poetic examples to explore:

- "Variation on the Word Sleep" by Margaret Atwood

- "Lullaby" by W.H. Auden

- "Wyknen, Blynken, and Nod" by Eugene Field

- "To Sleep" by John Keats

- "To Say Before Going to Sleep" by Rainier Maria Rilke

Good Night Throughout the World

Language is a lens through which we perceive and understand our experience of life, including how we frame and relate to sleep. For example, in English, we often say "go to sleep" as if the Land of Nod exists in another place to which we travel. Another popular term — that actually dates to the late fourteenth century — is "falling asleep"; it seems to infer that we succumb to the soporific state, or perhaps that we see it as some sort of descent. A tour of expressions in other languages can offer us a cross-cultural context for how sleep is perceived. Below you'll find sleep-encouraging idioms used in a variety of different languages and their literal translations. (Phonetic representations are used for languages that feature an alphabet other than Roman.)

- **Chinese:** *Jiāo jié* = To close one's eyes
- **Dutch:** *Slaap lekker* = Sleep tasty
- **Hebrew:** *Halomet paz* = Peaceful dreams
- **Hindi:** *Neend aa rahee hai* = Sleep is coming to me
- **Italian:** *Andiamo a nanna* = Let's go beddy-bye
- **Swahili:** *Lala salama* = Sleep safely

conventional illumination emits a type of light that curtails the production of the sleep-encouraging hormone melatonin, with research linking excessive light at night (known as LAN) to reduced sleep quality.

All said, there's no need to feel resigned that regularly getting a good night's sleep — and the well-being that comes with it — is out of your reach, or even inaccessible without medication or expensive gadgets. In fact, if you're someone who has sleep challenges, there are many things you can do to access more shut-eye. In the following chapter, we'll explore sleep-hygiene practices and self-care strategies; these can restore your restfulness, inspiring your ability to sleep well, so that you can enhance your physical and emotional well-being — including through your ability to connect to your dreams.

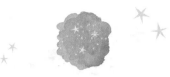

CHAPTER TWO

ENHANCING SLEEP

As mentioned in the last chapter, there is a wellspring of techniques and strategies that can be beneficial in transforming our relationship to rest. These can be helpful in amplifying our well-being in a more holistic and integrative way. Some of these are derived from an approach known as sleep hygiene, while others are integrative lifestyle practices that can help inspire relaxation. As you will see, there are numerous possibilities to explore, allowing you the freedom to find ones that appeal to your individual interests and address the underlying factors that keep you from a good night's sleep.

Sleep Hygiene

As the sleep loss epidemic has escalated, there's been a growing interest in a branch of health promotion specifically designed to champion habits that support better sleep. And while it may not have the sexiest of names — it's called sleep hygiene — its efficacy has resulted in it gaining significant recognition for the numerous benefits it accords. The term *sleep hygiene* was coined by one of the fathers of sleep medicine, Nathaniel Kleitman, in his 1939 book *Sleep and Wakefulness*; it was further codified as a health-promotion system in the 1970s by psychologist Peter Hauri. Today, it's an integral part of an approach to sleep medicine called Cognitive Behavioral Therapy for Insomnia (CBT-I for short). Owing to its demonstrated success, CBT-I has been recognized by both the U.S. National Institutes of Health and the American Academy of Sleep Medicine as an approach that can help those with insomnia disorder. If severe insomnia plagues you, you may want to look for a licensed health-care practitioner skilled in this practice. If you have challenges here and there in getting a good night's sleep, though, trying out some foundational sleep-hygiene principles on your own may do the trick. They may help transform sleep from your adversary into your ally. Here are some core principles of the sleep-hygiene approach.

REVERE SLEEP

See sleep for the exceptional worth and value that it has. Remember how important it is to your physical and emotional health (including your connection to your dreams). Elevate it from being a second-rate citizen of your life, forgoing any inclinations to be a card-carrying member of the "I'll sleep when I'm dead" club. If you prize it, you will more readily be able to prioritize it.

BEDS ARE FOR SLEEPING, DREAMING, AND SEX

A core sleep-hygiene principle is to only think of your bed as a place for sleeping, dreaming, and sex. We should see our bed as a haven, a place dedicated to these intimate and cherished experiences. If, instead, we view our beds as locations where we can do anything — catch up on social media, chat with our friends, watch television, and engage in other waking-life activities — we'll weaken the association that it holds with our sleep; this can impede upon our natural ability to drift off into cherished slumber once we're tucked in. Given that these other activities may be rousing and irritating, it may have us associate our bed as a site of struggle, and therefore a place that we don't feel at peace.

DON'T TOSS AND TURN IN BED

If we're beset with a bout of insomnia, sleep-hygiene professionals suggest that we get out of bed and go to another location to engage in a relaxing activity that may lull us back to sleep. The rationale for this is as follows: if you're tossing and turning, you'll see your bed as a place of strife, rather than of tranquility. Also, if you do find yourself waking up in the middle of the night, try not to stress about it. Getting agitated may only make it worse, kick-starting a cascade of stress hormones that will further keep you from feeling peaceful.

MAINTAIN A REGULAR SLEEP SCHEDULE

Try to have your bedtime be as consistent as possible, since this will allow your body to get into a regular groove when it comes to knowing when to sleep and when to awaken. To determine this time, calculate how much sleep you need (see page 28 for general guidelines) and at what hour you need to awaken; make sure to also build in extra time to wind down and fall asleep, as well as linger in bed in the morning so that you can connect to your dreams.

AVOID NAPS

If you regularly nap but then find you can't sleep well, restrain from your midday slumber for a week and see if this is helpful. While napping can be a luxurious experience, it can also impede upon our ability to fall asleep, since it reduces our "sleep pressure" (a biological response that encourages us to do so), keeping us awake past the time we want to doze off.

CREATE A SLEEP-INSPIRING ENVIRONMENT

Make your bedroom a place in which you feel relaxed. Encourage sleep by having the room be around 65°F (18°C), which is suggested to be a slumber-supportive temperature. Have it be as dark as possible at night, while also exposing yourself to lots of bright natural light when you awaken. You can find more suggestions for transforming your bedroom into a sanctuary in chapter 4.

AVOID EATING TOO CLOSE TO BEDTIME

Try to have your last meal hours before you go to sleep, so that your body won't be busy digesting when you're trying to power down. Also consider limiting or avoiding

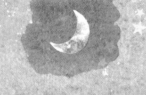

Normal Sleep Now Wasn't Normal Back Then

While we currently define good sleep as getting 7 or so uninterrupted hours, this wasn't always the case. Before the nineteenth century, segmented sleep was the norm, as documented by researcher A. Roger Ekirch in his book *At Day's Close: Night in Times Past*. People would sleep for several hours, called "first sleep," and then be awake for 1 to 2 hours. Then they would go back to sleep for several hours, called "second sleep." The span between the two sleep periods was referred to as "the watch," and was generally a time for reflection, dream-pondering, and sex (and sometimes even gathering with neighbors). So, if you find yourself getting up in the middle of the night for a bit, it may not be as abnormal as you might think. Just adjust your sleep time to accord for it, and enjoy this reflective watch period.

slower-to-digest foods — like meats and high-fat fare — at dinner. Additionally, try to steer clear of spicy foods close to bedtime; not only can they possibly cause heartburn, but they also may elevate your body temperature, which goes against the tide of the cooling necessary to promote sleepiness.

BE DISCERNING WITH BEVERAGES

Since caffeine has an average half-life of 5 hours (the amount of time it takes for 50 percent to be cleared from your body), avoid consuming it after midday. Remember that it's not only coffee and tea that have caffeine, but chocolate as well. While alcohol may help lull us to sleep, it leads to disruptions in our slumber pattern over the entire night. Finally, stay well hydrated during the day by drinking an adequate supply of water, but limit your intake about an hour before bedtime so you can reduce the chance of disturbing your sleep for a middle-of-the-night sojourn to the bathroom.

EXERCISE, BUT AT CERTAIN TIMES

Regular exercise promotes good sleep when done earlier in the day. Traditional sleep-hygiene recommendations suggest avoiding exercising hours before slumber, given that working out, notably in a high-intensity fashion, stimulates endorphins, as well as the sympathetic nervous system. Recent research differs, though, noting that non-high-impact exercise may not detract from drifting off. Connect to your personal experience to know what's best for you. If you find yourself challenged to sleep and you exercise in the late afternoon or evening, change up your fitness schedule and see if it makes a difference.

RELAX AND UNWIND

Begin to wind down a couple of hours before bedtime. Do some light stretches, take a bath, read a book that's inspiring and not agitating, and/or write in your journal. Dimming the lights or using candles a few hours before bedtime not only creates a calming environment but is also a melatonin-enhancing strategy (melatonin is a hormone that helps us slide into sleep).

LIMIT ELECTRONICS

While this one may be challenging in today's world, try to avoid being online an hour or so before bedtime. This can help limit your access to information that can be triggering or unnerving. Plus, avoiding your devices can curb your exposure to melatonin-depleting light. That said, if you'd rather not opt for a printed book over a digital one, or swap perusing photos on Instagram for those in magazines, make sure your phone, tablet, or computer has a blue-light-blocking screen filter. Or use a pair of blue-light-blocking glasses at night.

Self-Care Practices

There are many self-care practices that can help us to relax, reducing the tension we feel and allowing our nervous system to claim a restored sense of balance. Many of these practices not only have long histories of use, but they have also recently garnered support from the medical community, owing to research that demonstrates their benefits. (There are also a host of natural remedies — including herbs, essential oils, and flower essences — that can help you relax and invite in sleep, details about which you can find in chapter 3.)

MEDITATION AND MINDFULNESS

Numerous studies have found that meditation and mindfulness practices are associated with better sleep and may help people who struggle with insomnia. Why? While the reasons haven't been fully determined, it's thought to be related to the greater level of emotional resilience and diminished stress response that they offer. In fact, mindfulness practices have been shown to lower levels of cortisol, which is important because higher levels of this stress hormone have been linked with greater rates of insomnia. Once solely associated with spiritual traditions, there are now popular meditation and mindfulness practices that have a more secular bent.

In mindfulness, we work toward letting go and accepting. We find a way of perceiving that is unattached and equanimous; both our inner judge and the racing mind that often accompanies it become quiet, and we find ourselves filled with more calm and quietude. And with this shift in mental orientation, there is a concomitant adjustment in physiological factors, which seem to include both stress and inflammation reduction. Research has shown that those who are more apt to engage in repetitive thought processing, the experience in which our thinking gets stuck going back over the same notion again and again, have compromised sleep quality. Mindfulness practices help to create concentration and inspire intentional focus, reducing repetitive merry-go-round thinking.

Even if you feel that your busy schedule doesn't allow you the time for a regular meditation practice, you can still benefit by taking relaxing "mindful time-outs." For example, Take 5! — by just taking 5 minutes each day to close your eyes and mindfully concentrate on your breath, you'll have a direct route to experiencing more tranquility and relaxation. You can even do this mini-meditation practice without closing your eyes; for example, when you're in line at the supermarket, waiting for an elevator, sitting in traffic, or even doing the dishes, pay attention to your breath and see how this begins to ease your mind. You can also inspire inner calm by practicing mindful eating, in which you concentrate without distractions when you enjoy your meals, savoring each bite.

In addition to stillness-oriented meditation, there are mindfulness practices that incorporate movement, which have been found to offer sleep-supportive benefits. These include activities such as hatha yoga, tai chi, and qi gong, all of which have been found to improve sleep quality and/or reduce the severity of insomnia. While yoga may be familiar to many people, for its optimal slumber-supporting benefits, it's important to connect with your breath when you're practicing it. Tai chi is a style of martial arts known for its calm and integrated movements. Qi gong is a practice that coordinates breathing and meditative focus with a series of body postures.

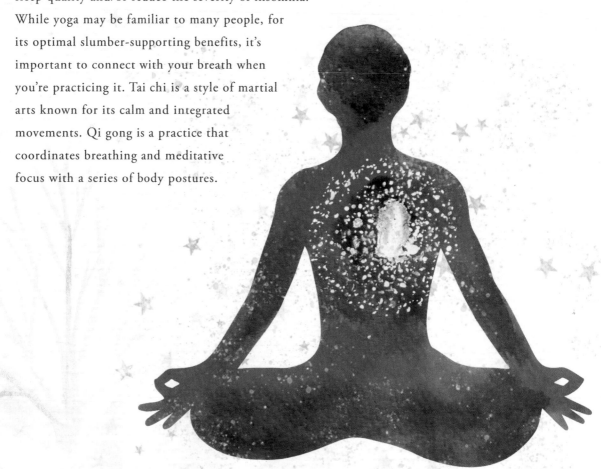

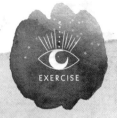

How to Meditate

Here's a simple way to meditate:

1 Maintain a comfortable position. Some people like to sit cross-legged on the floor on a bolster or pillow. Others prefer to sit in a chair. Use any props you need to help your body feel supported. Try to keep your spine as straight as possible. If sitting doesn't work for you, by all means lie down on the floor, placing a rolled-up towel under your knees if that feels more comfortable.

2 Close your eyes. Breathe naturally and notice your breath. If your mind wanders, just return your attention to your breath. Importantly, don't judge yourself if your mind starts to chatter and you forget to mind your breath. It's OK; just return to feeling and observing it.

3 Some people find it helpful to think the word *inhale* when they breathe in and *exhale* when they breathe out. Others like to say a mantra or word each time they inhale and exhale. Do what feels best for you.

4 Start off doing this practice for 10 minutes, building up to 20 minutes or more.

BREATHING PRACTICES

Slow and focused breathing techniques have been found to be calming to the central nervous system by enhancing parasympathetic activity, which helps us recover from stress. This calming has transformative value during the day, including helping us to prepare for deeper sleep. This suggestion comes not only from traditional health systems that feature breathwork, but also from modern scientific research. For example, one study found that 20 minutes of slow breathing helped improve sleep: people fell asleep faster, woke up less

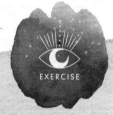

EXERCISE

The "365" Method

This is an approach that some health-care practitioners recommend for reducing stress and anxiety. Its benefits may extend to better sleep. The 365 signifies:

- Do the practice 3 times a day.

- Take 6 full breaths each minute: five-second inhales through your nose and five-second exhales through your mouth.

- Do this for 5 minutes. (Ideally, do this practice every day.)

frequently, and were able to get back to sleep more rapidly if they happened to wake up in the night. And speaking of somnambulist benefits, another study found that diaphragmatic breathing helps to reduce the production of cortisol and promote levels of melatonin.

On these pages are two easy-to-do breathwork practices to try. You can do them any time during the day, including right before bed.

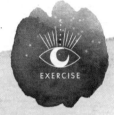

EXERCISE

The "4-7-8" Method

This technique is thought to be very relaxing, with many people saying that it is helpful in lulling them to sleep. (Since children's respiration rates are different than those of adults, this sequencing may not work best for them. For a child-friendly breathing practice, see page 207.) The 4-7-8 signifies:

- Inhale through your mouth for 4 counts.
- Hold your breath for 7 counts.
- Exhale through your mouth for 8 counts.

RELAXATION PRACTICES

In addition to mindfulness and breathing practices, there are a handful of other easy-to-do relaxation practices that may aid you in getting good sleep.

Yoga Nidra

Yoga nidra is a form of guided relaxation practice. Rooted in the yogic tradition, it is a technique that allows you to reach a very deep state of relaxation. It galvanizes a heightened awareness of your inner state, helping you to access a consciousness of quietude that can serve as a bridge to sleep. It does so through numerous mechanisms, including bringing your attention gently and habitually to various parts of the body in a way that allows you to withdraw your attention from them altogether. Research has suggested it has calming properties, able to reduce stress and anxiety. Also known as yogic sleep, it is thought to be helpful for those who struggle with slumber. Resources that can help you practice yoga nidra include online guided meditations or classes that may be offered at your local yoga studio or wellness center.

Hot Baths

Taking a bath about 90 minutes before bedtime may inspire sleep. Not only is the practice itself relaxing, but the warm temperature serves as a soporific signal. While you'll heat up in the bath, when you get out, your body will work to reduce your core temperature; given that reduced body heat is a prerequisite for the sleep cascade to unfold, this will help you to wind down into slumber. If you don't have a bathtub, or you're inclined to reduce your water consumption, opt for a 20-minute footbath instead; studies have shown it to have similar benefits. Make your bath more relaxing by turning off or dimming the lights and using candles. Play gentle music or use a pink noise machine to block out ambient sounds. Add 2 cups (475 ml) of Epsom salts and your favorite essential oils (use ½ cup [120 ml]) of salts if taking a footbath). You can also add some calming fragrance to your environment by using essential oils in an aromatherapy diffuser.

Progressive Muscle Relaxation

This technique, developed in the early twentieth century by physician Edmund Jacobson, is a practice in which you tense and then subsequently relax muscles throughout your body. It has been shown to be of value in treating insomnia. The benefits may come through both the tension release it affords, and how it engages you to focus your mind on something other than the thoughts that are streaming through. Do this relaxation practice in the evening to wind down. The whole process should take about 15 minutes. If you find it challenging to do on your own, look for recordings that will lead you through the process. Or get guidance from a skilled health-care practitioner trained in this method. To do the practice:

1   Lie down in a comfortable position.

2   Starting with your hands, clench them for about 5 seconds, and then relax them for 10 seconds before moving on to doing so in the next part of the body upon which you're focusing.

3   While different practitioners may suggest a different sequence, one common order is as follows: hands, lower arms, upper arms, shoulders, forehead, eyes and cheeks, mouth and jaw, neck, chest, back, stomach, hips and buttocks, thighs, lower legs, and feet.

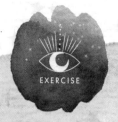

EXERCISE

Autogenic Training

Autogenic training is a self-guided relaxation technique that involves passive concentration. It was developed in the early twentieth century by psychiatrist Johannes Heinrich Schultz. Several research studies suggest that it not only plays an important role in stress management, but that it can also improve sleep patterns. It has been shown to help people fall asleep quicker and return to sleep more effortlessly should they have mid-sleep awakenings. Do this practice in the evening, as you're winding down near bedtime. Practitioners teach autogenic training in a sequential manner, having people concentrate on one of the phases for a short stretch of time before adding another. To do this practice, first find a comfortable position, whether sitting or lying down, and then begin to breathe in a rhythmic, even fashion. From there:

<u>1</u> Focusing on your arms, say to yourself several times that your arms are very heavy, as you notice this sensation. Follow this with saying that you are completely calm.

<u>2</u> Focusing again on your arms, say to yourself several times that your arms are warm, as you notice this sensation. Follow this with saying that you are completely calm.

3 Continue by focusing on your legs, applying the same approach as you did for your arms in steps 1 and 2.

4 Then focus on your heart, noting to yourself several times that your heartbeat is calm and regular as you notice this sensation. Follow this with saying that you are completely calm.

5 Now focus on your breath, noting to yourself several times that it is calm and regular, as you notice this sensation. Follow this with saying that you are completely calm.

6 Then focus on your abdomen, noting to yourself several times that it is warm, as you notice this sensation. Follow this with saying that you are completely calm.

7 Finally, focus on your forehead, noting to yourself several times that it is cool, as you notice this sensation. Follow this with saying that you are completely calm.

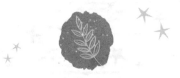

CHAPTER THREE

NATURAL REMEDIES FOR SLEEP

Nature's apothecary offers us an array of healing remedies that serve as powerful allies in our quest for well-being, including those that help us relax and invite in slumber. Here's a guide to herbs, essential oils, and flower essences that may inspire better sleep.

Herbal Teas

44

Consuming botanicals for well-being is definitely not a new tradition; in fact, it's one that spans across history and cultures. The oldest known compendium of herbs dates back to approximately 3000 BCE, and plant medicines have been used ever since in healing traditions the world over. Botanical medicine has become exceptionally popular over the past decades, widely available not only in a variety of stores, but also recommended by natural and conventional health-care practitioners alike. Some of the well-regarded relaxation-inspiring herbs include the ones below.

German Chamomile

An herbal remedy used for thousands of years, including for its sleep-promoting effects, its small flowers have a sweet, apple-like scent. Research has shown it to have sedative properties.

Hops

Well known for being an ingredient in beer, hops have been revered for their sleep-inducing as well as calming properties. The standard-bearer *Commission E Monographs* recognizes their use for addressing restlessness and sleep disturbances.

Lavender

With a research-supported stellar reputation for its calming properties, lavender has also been found to benefit sleep; the *Commission E Monographs* lists it as an approved botanical for restlessness and insomnia.

Lemon Balm

Also known as melissa, lemon balm has anti-stress properties, and is included in many pharmacopeias for its sleep-promoting ability. As it grows wild in many gardens, it may make an easily accessible and low-cost sleep aid.

Passionflower

Its use as a sleep tonic goes far back, first documented when Spanish explorers discovered the Aztecs using it for this purpose. It has been found to increase levels of the neurotransmitter GABA, which may account for some of its relaxing properties.

Valerian Root

One of the best-researched herbs for sleep disturbances, valerian was recommended for this benefit as far back as the second century CE by the esteemed physician Galen. It's often combined with other soporific herbs, such as passionflower and hops.

HOW TO USE HERBS

While herbs are available in tincture and capsule forms, making an herbal tea can be lovely. After all, the ritual of drinking something warm before bed can be very relaxing in and of itself. Ready-made tea bags are often a convenient way to enjoy a cup of tea. And yet, you may find that there are times when making your own with loose herbs elevates the ritual experience. To do so, you can either add them to a muslin tea sachet, or use a bamboo or metal tea strainer. In general, add 1 tablespoon of fresh herbs to 1 cup (240 ml) of boiling water and steep for about 5 minutes. The only exception is valerian; since you're using the root part, it takes longer to diffuse, about 10 minutes. Speaking of valerian, as it doesn't have the most endearing of fragrances, you may want to add other herbs to the mix when making a tea from it.

NOTE: As with all herbs, check with your health-care practitioner before using these to make sure none are contraindicated with any medicines you are taking or any health conditions you have.

Essential Oils

Aromatherapy is a holistic healing art that uses essential oils, aromatic concentrates distilled from the flowers, roots, fruit peels, barks, and resins of plants and trees. Different fragrances have unique properties, including their ability to inspire distinct feeling states; when we consider that the olfactory centers are directly related to our limbic system, a part of the brain associated with our emotions, the ability of scents to inspire different moods makes sense. The best way to enjoy aromatherapy is by using high-quality natural essential oils; synthetic versions of fragrances do not offer the same benefits.

ESSENTIAL OILS TO CONSIDER

Here are several essential oils that may inspire your sleep. Since scent is a personal preference, smell different ones — and the same one from different companies — to determine those that best resonate with you. (Find ways to keep your essential oils at hand, yet at the same time out of the reach of young children and pets.)

Bergamot
From the rind of the eponymous citrus fruit, bergamot essential oil has a joy-inspiring scent that can be quite centering.

Clary Sage
With its sweet and euphoric fragrance, clary sage may be of particular interest to women whose sleep disturbances are related to the sway of their hormones.

Damask Rose
While damask rose is on the more expensive side, the luxurious fragrance from this exquisite flower may help promote better sleep quality.

German Chamomile
This oil, from the flower that is well known for its calming tea, has a blue color and a soothing yet uplifting scent.

Jatamansi
Also known as spikenard, jatamansi, when diluted with massage oil and rubbed on the feet, is said to promote nighttime relaxation and curb insomnia.

Lavender

This popular oil has stress-reducing properties, may elevate melatonin levels, and has been found to enhance sleep quality.

Ylang Ylang

An essential oil that has a sultry and buoying scent, ylang ylang is thought to reduce tension, with people noting it inspires a more positive outlook on life.

HOW TO USE ESSENTIAL OILS

There are various ways of using essential oils, including:

Topically

Add several drops of essential oil to a carrier oil, such as one made from almond, jojoba, apricot kernel, or your favorite type. While this can be used for massage or moisturizing, it's also the best way to apply most essential oils. That's because the oils are so concentrated and may cause sensitivity reactions if applied directly to the skin in an undiluted fashion.

In the Bath

Place some Epsom salts in your hand and add a few drops of essential oil to it. Mix together and then add to bathwater. The salts will help the oil disperse in the water.

In a Mist

Add 12 drops of an essential oil to a 1-ounce (30-ml) glass bottle that features a mister top. Fill with filtered water. Shake before using and spritz your body or environment as desired.

In a Diffuser

Diffusers are devices that disperse small droplets of essential oils in the air to fragrance a room. You can also get diffusers that can aromatize your car.

Flower Essences

While flower essences are also derived from botanicals, unlike essential oils, they have no fragrance. Rather, they are natural elixirs made from flower-infused water, which work on an energetic level to restore mental and emotional balance. Each one addresses different personality characteristics and/or unique constitutional temperaments. While there are likely thousands of different flower essences, many people are introduced to this system of healing through the use of a popular formula of five Bach flowers, known as Rescue Remedy™, that is used to alleviate acute stress. There are numerous flower essences that may inspire sleep, each targeting a different underlying reason that may be keeping us from the Land of Nod. These include the following.

Aspen

There are times when worry keeps us tossing and turning, and yet we can't quite pin down the source of our disquietude. If it's hard to fall asleep because of a vague sense of dread and fear — the cause of which seems diffuse and not readily identifiable — consider Aspen flower essence.

Mimulus

If you're readily able to zero in on the cause of the fear and upset that's keeping you from getting your forty winks — whether it's a thunderstorm, tomorrow's staff meeting, a health concern, or something else recognizable — consider Mimulus flower essence.

Red Chestnut

If you need some compassionate detachment because you're finding yourself staying up at night worrying about something for someone else — whether it's your partner's job security, your aging parent's health, or the current whereabouts of your teenager — consider Red Chestnut flower essence.

Vervain

There are times when a day of adventure and possibility still has us so revved up when we hit the pillow that we feel too overexcited to sleep. If an abundance of enthusiasm for something in your life has you wound up and you want to wind down, consider Vervain flower essence.

White Chestnut

That racing mind? Those merry-go-round thoughts? While they can take us off our A game during the day, they can also create a barrier that keeps us from falling asleep. If you want a way to center and calm your chattering mind, consider White Chestnut flower essence.

HOW TO USE FLOWER ESSENCES

Flower essences can be used either orally or topically. If you want to use them orally, the recommended dosage is usually four drops of each essence four times a day. You can take them straight from their container, add them to a cup of water, or put them in a glass dropper bottle filled with filtered water. Diluting a flower essence in water will not dilute its potency. Most flower essences are made in a base of alcohol, so take this into consideration if you are alcohol-sensitive or you're giving them to children; you may be able to find ones that are instead made with a glycerin base. If you want to use the flower essences topically, you can apply them to your skin or add them to a bath. You can also place four drops of each in a mister bottle filled with water (and an essential oil, if you'd like) and spritz yourself or your environment several times each day. Flower essences can be purchased at holistic pharmacies, natural food stores, or through natural health practitioners who work with these healing agents.

CHAPTER FOUR

CREATING A SLEEP AND DREAM SANCTUARY

Our bedroom is our most personal and private haven, a space in which we relax and let go, enjoying experiences that are nourishing for our body, mind, and soul. It's the room in which we undertake two of the activities that can powerfully promote our well-being: sleeping and dreaming. And it's also the place in our home in which we generally spend the most time: if you sleep 7 to 8 hours each night, you spend about one-third of your life in your bedroom. Treating it as a sanctuary, a place we cherish and revere, can help us sleep and dream even better. And while our attitudes toward our bedroom can go a long way in terms of elevating its sanctity, there are also practical design steps we can take to help us create a more salutary space that promotes relaxation and well-being. In this chapter, you'll learn some design principles that can enhance your bedroom's energy and flow, how to create a dream altar, and the slumber-inspiring importance of environmental factors such as light, temperature, air quality, and sound.

Bedroom Design Principles

We want to design our bedrooms so that they are as beautiful and comfortable as possible. Additionally, we also want them to emanate a sense of ease and inspire relaxation. To help toward this aim, we can turn to feng shui, the ancient Chinese art of furniture placement and design that is popular today. It offers valuable tips on how to arrange furnishings to allow for energy to more effortlessly flow and peacefulness to feel as if it's streaming throughout. According to feng shui, the bedroom is the most important room in the house, so arranging it thoughtfully is of great value. Here are some feng shui design principles that can infuse your bedroom with more of a sanctuary feel:

- Remove anything that isn't meaningful and doesn't promote ease and relaxation. The letter from your ex that's stored in your nightstand drawer? That old, frayed, beaten-up chair? The plant that's on its last leg? Move them to another room if you don't want to remove them altogether.

- Avoid mirrors within the sightline of the bed; as they reflect light, mirrors are thought to amplify the energy in the room, which may interfere with the calming feel that we want our bedroom to have.

- Be thoughtful about the artwork you choose, having it be of images that represent what you want to manifest in your life.

- If the ceiling has overhead beams, avoid having furniture such as chairs or your bed under them, or perhaps cover the beams with draping.

Seven Sleep and Dream Sanctuary Guidelines

1 Think of your bed as a place dedicated to enjoying some of life's most intimate and soul-enriching experiences: sleeping, dreaming, and lovemaking.

2 Treat your bedroom as a comforting haven where you can find peace and solace.

3 Design your bedroom so it helps you to naturally unwind when you spend time there.

4 Don't bring work — nor other things that activate or agitate your mind — into the bedroom.

5 If you need to have a stirring conversation with your partner or child, opt to do it in another room.

6 Make your bed each morning. Having a tidy and fresh bed into which you can climb each night helps to further invite in restful sleep.

7 If possible, have your bedroom be a tech-free zone, keeping computers, tablets, and even the television in another room.

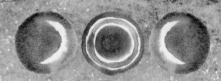

The Bedroom Throughout History

Like most everything, the bedroom has taken on evolving roles depending upon the current culture's needs. It's only been relatively recently that bedrooms have become the private enclaves that they now are. Previously, many families slept in a common room, not only out of economic need but also as a way to foster a sense of community and protect from possible middle-of-the-night intruders. Bedrooms were also public stages where the affairs of life were conducted. It was in this room that many of life's significant activities would take place: weddings, socializing, business deals, births, and deaths. Beds were prized items; rather expensive — even more so than by today's standards — they were status symbols, passed down from generation to generation, and often items included in wills. Today, bedrooms have evolved to reflect the current cultural context and the needs of their denizens. They may serve as playrooms for kids, hideaways and study spaces for teenagers, offices for gig worker...and ideally, a place where we all open to the rejuvenation that comes with our sleep and dreams.

- If possible, don't have a bookshelf in the bedroom, since it enhances the active energy of the room. If, owing to space constraints, you do need to have one in there, arrange the books horizontally rather than vertically, to avoid the room's energy feeling as if it's being spliced.

- According to feng shui, neutral and light tranquil colors are better for bedrooms than bright or deep colors like red, orange, purple, and black.

- While it may be ideal to not have a television in your bedroom, if you do have one, position a screen that blocks it from sight when you're sleeping. Or put it in an armoire with a door.

- As best as possible, hide all electrical cords.

- If you need to have gym or office equipment in your bedroom, cover it with a beautiful piece of fabric or obscure it with a screen when it's not in use.

THE BED

Owing to the bed being the centerpiece of the bedroom and the important role it has, feng shui offers numerous principles related to its optimal positioning. It's suggested that the bed should be located in what's known as the "commanding position." In this placement, the bed would be facing the door so that you could readily see it and anyone who enters or exits the room. However, you don't necessarily want it to be exactly in line with the door, as you want to avoid having your feet pointing directly toward it. The head of the bed should ideally be against a solid wall. If the wall behind you has a window, try to alleviate any potential drafts, and also be sure to draw the curtains at night. It's thought best to not hang art over the bed. And try to also avoid placing the head of your bed in a position that has it sharing a wall with the bathroom, notably the one on which the toilet is located. (And speaking of your bathroom, ideally, you shouldn't be able to see it from the bed; if that's unavoidable, remember to keep the door shut.) Solid headboards are thought to provide more stability than those that have slats. The headboard should be positioned so that it's stable and doesn't wobble. You should ideally have space on three sides of the bed, so that there's easy ingress into and out of it. It's not only a practical idea, but one thought to promote more optimal energy circulation.

THE MATTRESS

As we spend about one-third of our life in bed, it makes sense to prioritize having a good mattress. And while it can be a high-ticket item, if we think about how elemental sleep and dreams are to well-being, we can readily see how a good-quality mattress may be the piece of furniture that provides us with the best ROI. One of the premier roles that a good mattress has is to support the alignment of your spine. Not only will this have you be more comfortable and therefore sleep better, but it will also allow you to feel better during the day. It should encourage your spine to maintain a neutral position, with your lower back able to preserve its natural curve. As a general rule, mattresses last five to ten years. It's good to replace yours when it feels lumpy, you start waking up sore, or when you notice that you regularly feel better when sleeping elsewhere. That said, discomfort caused by sleeping isn't solely the realm of our mattress; if you wake up with neck or shoulder pain, it could be your pillow that's the culprit.

Choosing the Best Mattress and Pillow

We've come a long way since the original mattress, which dates back to 77,000 years ago and was composed of reeds covered by insect-repelling leaves. Technological advances have made it so that there are a host of different options — including inner spring, memory foam, hybrid, air-filled, and futons — from which to choose. Which one is best for you depends upon several factors, including your go-to sleep position, whether you run hot or cold at night, if you occupy the bed alone or with someone else, and, of course, your budget.

Also, don't forget about the value of having quality pillows; they play an essential role in promoting well-being by supporting your neck and helping your spine maintain a neutral position, warding off aches and pains that may otherwise occur. Pillow-purchasing considerations include: (1) its loft supports your sleeping style (stomach, side, or back); (2) whether you prefer it is made of natural or synthetic materials; (3) making sure you're not allergic to what it's filled with; and, (4) the price.

NIGHTSTANDS

Nightstands play an important role in the sleep and dream sanctuary. After all, they serve as an accessible resting spot for the items that give us comfort as we fall asleep and awaken — whether that's a glass of water, reading material, an alarm clock, or the like. Plus, their role in assisting us in our dreamwork is highly valuable. They are where we place the tools — such as paper and a writing instrument, or a recording device — through which we document our dream memories. From a feng shui perspective, like everything else in the bedroom, your nightstand should be orderly and clutter-free. If yours is overflowing with stuff, consider whether some of what you're keeping there can be stored elsewhere. Can your supplement bottles be kept in the bathroom? Can all but the current novel you're reading remain on a bookshelf? Can your ambient noise–reducing machine be placed on a bureau instead? If you do find that you need access to a variety of sundry items, arrange them thoughtfully on a beautiful tray or in decorative boxes, or get a nightstand that comes with drawers. Even if you sleep alone, feng shui principles still recommend that, space permitting, there be a nightstand on each side of the bed, since it will make the area feel more even and balanced. Nightstands with smoother, rather than sharp, edges are preferred.

CLEAR THE CLUTTER

From a feng shui perspective, clutter is not only messy, but it also represents unfinished business that may energetically drain us. It impedes vitality and restricts life from flowing forward. The first rule of bedroom decluttering is to take the things that you've stored under your bed and find a new spot for them. That's because we want the foundation upon which we sleep to be free-flowing, and not the storehouse for things such as books, shoes, or any non-treasured items we don't otherwise know where to keep. If limited space makes it a necessity to use the under-bed area for storage, dedicate it to keeping things that are softer and more neutral (like t-shirts, extra blankets, pillows, etc.). If your closet is in your bedroom, make sure it's in good order. Do a deep cleaning and keep it organized. And regardless of its state of order, keep the door to it closed when you're not using it. The same goes for cabinet drawers. Recently said goodbye to a lover with whom you shared the bed? Do a room clearing by burning sage or palo santo as a way to release their energy. Also, remove any of the things of theirs that you truly don't want around you anymore.

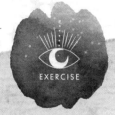

Creating a Dream Altar

Another way that you can transform your bedroom into a sanctuary is to create a dream altar, which can bring more intentionality to your oneiric practice. By doing so, you're creating a dedicated space that reminds you of the power of your dreams and your commitment to seeking the insights they provide. To do so, first find a place that works best for you, whether on a low table, a shelf, the top of your armoire, or even your nightstand. Have it feature items that have personal meaning and significance. To get you started thinking about designing yours, here are some ideas on what it can feature:

- Candles
- Flowers, whether fresh or dried
- Found objects like shells or sea glass
- Small pieces of art
- Photographs of meaningful places
- Pictures of spiritual teachers
- Iconographic figurines
- Tarot or angel cards
- Crystals
- Sacred texts
- Notes that reflect dream intentions
- Palo santo, sage, or incense for smudging

Dream Altar Tips

■ If you're practicing dream incubation (see chapter 11) and you want a spot to place a reminder of what creative problem you're trying to solve, you can also make space for it on your altar.

■ To heighten the intentionality of your dream altar, remember to do a clearing before you set it up and any time you feel it could use some energetic amplification. You can do this by using palo santo, sage, or your favorite incense.

■ When you're traveling, bring along some sacred items, so that you can create a dream altar wherever you are.

■ If you share your bedroom with a partner, you can each have your own altar. Or create one together.

■ See if your children are interested in having a dream altar in their room. While this may be something more aligned with older kids, it could also be an empowering strategy to help little ones who are struggling with nightmares, as they can put items on it that help them feel safe and protected.

Environmental Considerations

It's not just furniture that has an important function when it comes to our bedroom being a haven for a restful night's sleep. Paying attention to environmental factors such as light, temperature, air quality, and sound may also do wonders.

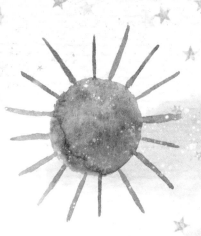

LIGHT

One of the keys to sleeping well and feeling refreshed during the day is modulating the light to which we are exposed. Much of the reason has to do with melatonin. This hormone plays an important role in regulating our circadian rhythms. Its release occurs with darkness, while light suppresses its production. Melatonin is one of the chemical signals in our brains that inspires the sleep cycle. And so, if we want our brains to shift into their somnolent state, having adequate amounts of melatonin is key.

As it turns out, blue light can disrupt sleep cycles, since it tells your body to stop producing melatonin. Therefore, be selective in the lights you use in your bedroom, avoiding certain LED and other bulbs known to feature it. Consider having your bedroom lights be on dimmers so that you can prevent them from being too bright before you go to sleep. Opt for lamps that shine light toward the ceiling rather than downward, as this, too, can create a more relaxed atmosphere. Other sources of blue light are the electrical devices we so readily rely upon in our modern lives. Therefore, avoid using your phone, tablet, and computer close to bedtime. If you can't readily do so, and need to use your tech devices while in bed, get some glasses that block the blue light, or use software programs that will modulate the spectrum of light that your gadgets emit.

If light streams in from outside, consider getting blackout curtains that will encourage there to be more darkness. If your bedroom just isn't dark enough for you, consider using an eye mask. Eliminate or reduce other sources of light; for example, avoid having a clock that has a bright digital readout. While night-lights may have kept us company when we were little kids, they aren't limited to use only by the young. In fact, they may still be helpful tools, allowing us to avoid turning on jarring brighter lights during middle-of-the-night journeys to the bathroom. Look for ones that have a red- or orange-hued bulb, as these will be less stimulating than those that emit the more blue-green light that's reflective of daytime.

As much as we want our bedrooms to be dark at night, we want them to be light in the morning. This helps inspire a feeling of alertness, while also signaling to our body that it should curb melatonin production. Open the curtains to let light filter in. Consider getting a sunrise alarm, one whose light gets gradually brighter in the morning as your wake-up time arrives. If it makes sense for you, get a smart lighting system that you can program to dim, go off, and then gradually go on at specified times.

TEMPERATURE

Temperature also plays a key role in helping us sleep, with thermoregulation integrally linked to our sleep and wake cycles. Our body temperature varies throughout the day, according to our naturally built-in circadian rhythms; it drops as bedtime approaches, with the lowest point being about 2 hours after we enter slumber. Researchers have found that our core body temperature needs to drop a bit to initiate our drifting off to sleep. As such, since the ambient climate of your bedroom can play a key role in lulling you to sleep, lowering it to a target temperature will help to reduce your basal temperature. It's thought that, for the average person, 65°F (18°C) is a good goal, with children and seniors needing it to be a few degrees warmer. If that temperature sounds cold, remember you can always add another layer of blankets to your bed. You can also keep warm upon arising with slippers and a robe accessible by your bedside.

Alternatively, if 65°F (18°C) sounds like an impossible dream in the summertime, or your bedroom heat retention is its gift in the winter but its curse other times of the year, there are temperature-reduction strategies you can employ. Get a fan to circulate the air, as that can make it appear cooler. Open the windows, if possible. You can also try cooling yourself by placing a cold gel pack in your pillowcase. Or, look for pillows made with more cooling fabrics, as well as specially designed mattress toppers that you can program to different temperatures.

AIR QUALITY

More and more research has shown that the air we breathe has significant impacts upon our health. And while we usually associate air pollution with the outdoors, it turns out that indoor air may actually be more contaminated. And while we may not be able to control the air quality of our workplaces or the commercial spots we frequent, we can do so in our homes. If we were going to choose one spot in which to concentrate our

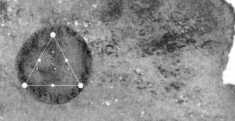

Electromagnetic Fields

Another environmental factor that may possibly have an impact upon our well-being is the presence of electromagnetic fields (EMFs). After all, given that our nervous system and heart operate via electrical signals, some people question whether being constantly surrounded by EMFs, including when we sleep, can have a deleterious effect upon our slumber and our health. At this point, most of the findings that suggest a purported impact of EMFs on health come from anecdotal evidence. The minimal research that has been done hasn't yet drawn a strong correlation. That said, if you feel you are hypersensitive to EMFs, or you just like the idea of fully turning off when your waking mind is turned off, there are some easy things you can do to reduce your exposure to EMFs in your bedroom. Don't sleep near circuit breakers. Shut the Wi-Fi off when you go to bed. Have your alarm clock be battery-operated. And if you keep your phone in your bedroom, switch it to airplane mode.

air-quality enhancing efforts, it seems that the bedroom would be a good place to start, given all the time we spend there. You may just find that doing so gives your well-being a boost, noticing that you have less congestion, low-level fatigue, brain fog...and, also, better sleep. Here are some tips to enhance your bedroom's air quality:

- Regularly clean your bedroom, including vacuuming the carpets or mopping the wood floors. Consider using nontoxic cleaners that are either fragrance-free or have scents derived from natural essential oils. This would include the detergent you use to clean your linens.

- Consider making the bedroom a shoe-free zone, so you don't bring in dirt from outside. Have slippers by the bedroom door that you can readily put on.

- Make sure your heating sources have good venting, with ducts that are regularly cleaned.

- Watch for water accumulation, to prevent the growth of mold spores.

- Consider getting an air filter to remove ambient pollutants.

Indoor Plants

Many plants are thought to act like natural filters, cleaning the air of pollutants such as formaldehyde, benzene, and carbon monoxide; but, while the research supporting this finding isn't yet conclusive, having plants in your bedroom may still be beneficial, as they breathe life into a space, both figuratively as well as literally, since they take in carbon dioxide and release oxygen. Plus, they add natural beauty and may have additional health benefits: research with hospital patients found that plants and flowers placed in their rooms helped reduce anxiety and lower blood pressure. Some of the plants often cited to help with air quality include golden pothos, spider plants, and peace lilies. If you want to infuse some natural fragrances into the room, notably those that are calming, you could consider a jasmine, gardenia, or lavender plant. From a feng shui perspective, corners are a great location for plants, since energy can otherwise stagnate in these spots. Of course, if you have small children or pets, ensure that the plants in which you're interested are not toxic to them. Also, if you have mold allergies, you may need to be more careful about having plants in the bedroom, as the soil may contain spores to which you could be sensitive.

SOUND

Some people can sleep through anything, while others awaken to a drop of a pin. If you're sound-sensitive, you want to do what you can to minimize any auditory interruptions that can disrupt your Zzzs. In addition to reducing background noise, there are also active measures you can adopt to help block your exposure to sounds. For some, earplugs readily do the trick. They come in a variety of shapes and materials — for example, silicone ones mold to your ears, while foam ones are pre-shaped. If you're into tech gadgets, you may want to look into noise-canceling headsets or earbuds. Another option to consider is getting a sleep sound machine. These play white noise or pink noise, the latter of which some people find to be more soothing, as it contains less high-frequency sounds. If you're someone who likes to fall asleep to calming music, program it so that it shuts off automatically after a certain point, so that it doesn't stir you to awaken in the middle of the night. Traveling? Ask for a quiet room — away from the elevator, busy streets, and ice machines — when making your reservation. Also, some hotels feature quiet zones or quiet rooms, so consider this as another quality to look for when researching for your travels.

PART II:

dreams

CHAPTER FIVE

THE DREAMING MIND

For all the virtue and value that people throughout history have accorded to dreams, and all the abundance of philosophical perspectives that scholars have held about them, what exactly occurs in the mind when we're dreaming was terra incognita for millennia. Still, there had been somewhat of a consensus that as animated as oneiric visions can be, that when we are sleeping and dreaming, the mind is downregulated and relatively asleep. That all changed in 1953, when a groundbreaking paper was published in the journal *Science* that would forever transform our understanding. In this article, entitled "Regularly Occurring Periods of Eye Motility, and Concomitant Phenomena, During Sleep," the authors, Eugene Aserinsky and Nathaniel Kleitman, reported on the discovery of rapid eye movement (REM) sleep that they had uncovered during research that transpired in the previous two years.

The experiments — which then research assistant Aserinsky conducted in Kleitman's sleep lab at the University of Chicago — and their subsequent reporting laid the groundwork for future seminal sleep and dream discoveries. These expounded on how REM sleep — which we now know accounts for about 25 percent of the total time adults spend sleeping — is the period believed to be when the most vivid dreams occur. They also discovered that, in addition to the occurrence of the rapid eye movements under closed lids, which became the hallmark of this period, other physiological shifts transpire in REM, such as increased heart and respiratory rates. And, strikingly, it was also then shown that while we may be sleeping during REM, the brain is actually not, with brain waves looking relatively similar to those present during waking. The seemingly anomalous occurrence of an awake mind with a sleeping body inspired French neuroscientist Michel Jouvet to coin "paradoxical sleep" as an alternative term for REM.

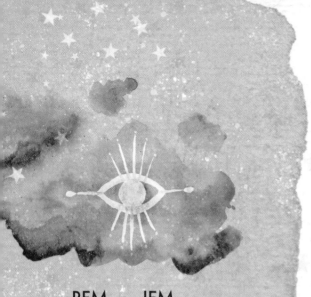

REM vs. JEM

If you think that rapid eye movement and REM aren't the most poetic of names for the period of sleep in which the most poetic of events — vivid dreams — occur, it could have been worse. Eugene Aserinsky has shared that REM wasn't his original choice; owing to the abrupt movements that he noticed the eyes making during this period, he first thought to call it jerky-eye movement sleep (JEM).

Sleep and Dream Stages

Since the discovery of REM, sleep was recategorized into having two main periods: that which features rapid eye movements, and that which does not. The former, of course, is known as REM sleep. The latter is known by a term that reflects not so much what it is, but what it isn't: it is known as non-REM (or NREM) sleep. NREM sleep begins when we first fall asleep and features three distinct parts, known as stage 1, stage 2, and stage 3. REM sleep begins after these have initially appeared, and is sometimes referred to as stage 4 sleep. Here are some more details on the features of each.

NREM SLEEP

Stage 1

This is the transitional state of drowsiness we enter when we first begin to fall asleep. It's a state of consciousness during which we can easily be awakened. High-frequency, low-amplitude beta waves in the brain, which are generally associated with engagement in mental activities, begin to be replaced by theta waves. We experience a slight decrease in muscle tone, and our response to external stimuli begins to shift.

Stage 2

During this stage, our body temperature decreases, as does our heart rate. Stage 2 is characterized by the appearance of brain wave forms known as sleep spindles and K complexes. There is further reduction in both muscle activity and conscious awareness of the environment. Stages 1 and 2 are considered light sleep.

Stage 3

Once divided into two different stages, this period of slow-wave sleep (SWS) is now considered as one. This is the time at which the deepest sleep occurs, and when it's the most difficult to awaken people from sleep. During SWS, our brain activity features a concentration of slow-speed delta waves. Our eyes are not moving, and there is continued reduction in muscle tone and responsiveness. This restorative stage of sleep is our time to get deep rest. It's also the period when growth hormone release increases, and our immune system becomes replenished. Sleepwalking, bedwetting, and night terrors occur in this phase.

A Powerful Trio

While Eugene Aserinsky and Nathaniel Kleitman are noted as co-authors of the famous *Science* article detailing the finding of REM, it was actually Aserinsky's work that formed the foundation of this discovery. With his persistent and innovative approach to research, he actually had one of his initial sleep-study breakthroughs when observing rapid eye movements during slumber in a most unusual, and familial, laboratory subject: his eight-year-old son Armond. Kleitman is considered the father of modern sleep research, establishing the first lab to study the workings of sleep at the University of Chicago. His contributions to the field are nothing short of monumental. In addition to co-authoring the now famous REM sleep-discovery study, he also wrote the influential 1939 book *Sleep and Wakefulness*; as we saw in chapter 2, it was in there that he coined the term *sleep hygiene*. After Aserinsky's initial discoveries, he was assisted by then-medical student William Dement, who had a strong interest in further understanding how REM was related to dreaming. Dement went on to not only make significant research advances, but also to author the seminal book *The Promise of Sleep*, as well as establish the first sleep clinic at Stanford University.

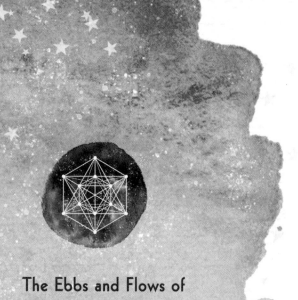

The Ebbs and Flows of NREM and REM

During sleep, our body maintains the integrity of its neural networks, which is vital for brain function, including emotional memory consolidation. During NREM, aspects of faulty neural networks are broken down, while their connections are re-strengthened during REM. While it's still not fully clear why this occurs as it does, this NREM/REM deconstruct-to-reconstruct partnership may underlie why the amount spent in each of these stages varies throughout the night.

REM SLEEP

Stage 4

While this is the fourth stage of sleeping, it's not usually referred to as stage 4, but just as REM. It's the period that's come to be most associated with dreams. And while researchers have discovered that dreams do occur in other sleep stages, something that they didn't realize until recently, it's still thought that it's in REM that we experience the most vivid of our oneiric visions.

SLEEP STAGE CYCLING

In addition to there being different stages of sleep, what's interesting is that there's a repeating rhythm to their occurrence. It's not that there's a single trajectory from stage 1 through REM that goes throughout the whole night. Rather, this four-stage cycle, through NREM and REM, usually lasts about 90 minutes (although it can be as long as 120 minutes) and repeats itself throughout our slumber. As such, if you get 8 hours of sleep, you're likely experiencing four or five full REM cycles, and consequently about four or five periods replete with vivid dream potential.

However, sleep stage cycling is even more nuanced than that, in a way that has significant repercussions for dreaming. As the subsequent 90-minute cycles occur, the time that each sleep stage occupies shifts.

For example, in the beginning of the night, deep and restful sleep (stage 3 SWS) takes up a big portion of each cycle. Yet, as the night turns to morning, its allocated time reduces, and more sleep is taken up by REM. This means that for some not-yet-identified reason, as we get closer to transporting ourselves back to waking, we spend a concentrated time in this stage in which graphic and memorable dreams occur. So, if you sleep 8 hours, and approximately one-quarter of your sleep is REM, then you'll have 2 hours each night in which you can have dreams that may be dynamic, animated, and evocative. Looked at another way, on average, one-twelfth of our day yields to us the potential to have powerful oneiric visions.

The Physiology of a Dreaming Brain

The dreaming brain is so fascinating and unique that many researchers contend that there are actually three primary brain states, or ways in which it fashions itself: the awake brain, the sleeping brain, and the dreaming brain. As previously discussed, there are similarities in brain wave activity between the dreaming REM state and the awake state. In addition, through EEG (electroencephalogram) testing, research has found that when an activity is undertaken while awake and while dreaming, the brain reveals a similar activation pattern. However, there are some notable differences between the dreaming REM brain and what is occurring while we're awake. The unique ways in which they express themselves may very well help us understand more about why oneiric visions appear as they do.

During REM, the brain area known as the prefrontal cortex (PFC) is downregulated. Given that it governs what's considered to be executive function, it controls such things as critical thinking, judgment, and self-control, all of which are tamped down during dreaming. The PFC is also thought to be involved in metacognition, the knowledge that you know that you have knowledge, the witness part of you that knows that you are thinking. When all of these functions aren't operating as they usually do in the waking state, we may then feel a more fluid sense of self that is able to expand beyond the boundaries of what's deemed acceptable and realistic, a quality we associate with our dreams. Plus, without metacognition, we can be experiencing something bizarre while lacking the rational judgment to denote that it's actually bizarre, a classic attribute of dreams. We don't know we are thinking, and invariably we then don't know we are dreaming.

That is, unless we are lucid dreaming, a state in which the PFC is not as passive as it is in regular dreaming, which may be why it's an experience filled with the awareness that you are actually dreaming. (You can find more information on lucid dreams in chapter 9.)

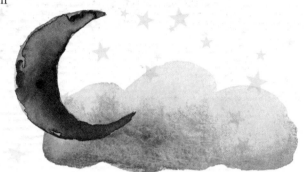

Other parts of the brain, though, exhibit an upregulation during REM dreaming. These include the limbic system, the seat of our emotional mind. Additionally, the part of our brain related to visual awareness is energized. This may help explain why dreams can have such a strong feeling tone, as well as why they are so graphic and pictorial. Additionally, certain brain chemicals appear in differing levels when we are dreaming compared to when we are awake. This includes the neurotransmitter norepinephrine, which is at a reduced level when we're dreaming; since one of its functions is to help shuttle short-term memories into long-term ones, this may be one of the reasons that it's so difficult to recall our dreams. (For more on dream recall, see chapter 12.)

Another hallmark of the REM stage is that most people (except those with REM disorders) experience muscle paralysis during it. Known as muscle atonia, it's thought to be a mechanism to protect us, so that we don't act out our dreams and potentially incur harm. What's also fascinating about the dreaming brain is that the images and feelings that it brings forth come not from processing the external world; after all, when we are sleeping, our eyes are closed and our senses aren't processing at the same level as when we are awake. Rather, it seems that most of the ingredients that the dreaming mind uses to create each unique oneiric journey come from within, from the deep recesses of the landscape of our consciousness.

Factors That Impact REM Dreams

There are some physiological factors that may actually deter vivid dreams from occurring as they usually do, owing to their ability to disturb our sleep architecture (the structural organization of our sleep) and cause REM disruption. This may manifest in either reducing our ability to have highly activated and memorable dreams, or in shifting sleep cycles in such a way that we have exceptionally animated dreams early in the morning. Disturbing regular REM cycles may have negative impacts upon our memory and emotional equilibrium in ways that have yet to be fully illuminated.

ALCOHOL

While alcohol may lull some people to sleep, it disrupts sleep architecture. It reduces the amount of REM we undergo during the first half of the night. But, in the body's natural attempt to maintain balance, it later creates what's known as REM rebound, in which we have lengthened periods of REM in the second half of sleep. This may account for people reporting more vivid dreams after having a few drinks. Yet, for others, this reduces their REM dream time by causing more frequent arousals while the body is working to eliminate the alcohol.

ANTICHOLERGENIC DRUGS

Anticholergenic drugs — those that function by blocking the action of the neurotransmitter acetylcholine — also reduce REM sleep. Numerous drugs have anticholergenic properties, including some used to treat overactive bladders, Parkinson's disease, allergies, and other conditions. That research has suggested that long-term use of anticholergenics may be linked to an increased risk of dementia has some researchers wondering even more about the role of REM in maintaining brain health.

ANTIDEPRESSANTS

Many antidepressant medications suppress REM sleep. These include those in the three major classes of such drugs: the monoamine oxidase inhibitors (MAOI), the tricyclic antidepressants (TCA), and the selective serotonin-reuptake inhibitors (SSRI).

CANNABIS

Preliminary research suggests that cannabis, as well as tetrahydrocannabinol (THC) edibles, reduces REM sleep. While cannabinoids (CBD) have been researched for their potential benefit in treating a condition called REM sleep behavior disorder, the effects of CBD on sleep stages and dreams are not fully known.

REM Sleep Behavior Disorder

Typically during REM sleep, our eyes are shut and our muscles tone is inactivated. This feels like nature's safeguard, so that we won't be stirred to act out the actions that animate our dreams. However, not everyone is so lucky. There's a condition called REM sleep behavior disorder (RBD) in which muscles don't disengage and sleep paralysis doesn't occur. This leads to dreamers often acting out their dreams both vocally and in movements that could be quite animated, and possibly dangerous. RBD occurs more frequently in those with narcolepsy, and many people who have Parkinson's disease and Lewy body dementia have RBD preceding their diagnosis. As such, it is thought to be a possible predictive factor for these conditions, although not everyone who has the condition will develop those neurodegenerative diseases. It is more common in the elderly than in younger people. While its causes are not fully understood, RBD may be related to damage in the part of the brain that controls muscle atonia (the loss of tone and strength) that naturally occurs during REM sleep. While usually chronic, there are some cases in which it is more acute, brought on by shifts in certain factors, including alcohol or drug withdrawal. For those with RBD, modifying their bedroom environment to minimize injury is a first-line strategy. There are some medications used to help mitigate the condition, with newer research suggesting that high-dose melatonin supplements may also be of benefit. Those with RBD should seek guidance from a trained health-care practitioner.

INSOMNIA

If you have the type of insomnia that has you waking up in the early morning hours, unable to fully go back to sleep, you may miss out on the extended REM sleep periods that occur during this time. Given these are when vivid dreams are likely to happen, this form of insomnia may not only rob you of your sleep, but also of the ability to have quite memorable dreams.

SLEEP APNEA

Non-treated sleep apnea occurs in both NREM and REM sleep, yet has been found to be more prevalent during the latter. This may be due to the reduction of muscle tone that is a characteristic of this sleep stage. Among its other consequences, the interrupted breathing that is a hallmark of non-treated sleep apnea may cause awakenings that fragment REM sleep periods.

CHAPTER SIX

DREAMING THROUGH LIFE

As we know, our dreams may change throughout our lives. Those that we have when we're adults are quite different than those we had as kids, or even teenagers. Seeing how dreams shift can give us fascinating insights into developmental psychology as well as the changing roles that they may play in our lives.

Infants

Given that infants don't readily have access to verbal language, it's uncertain what their dreams may be like. Of course, we do know that they spend a lot of time in REM sleep, approximately half of their entire sleep cycle (compared to about 25 percent for the average adult). This makes sense when we consider that this sleep stage is noted for its inherent importance to brain development. Whether they are experiencing the vivid dreams that occur in REM sleep, however, is currently unknown.

Early and Middle Childhood

Most research on children and dreams begins with those who are three or four years old, at which time many describe their dreams in a sentence or two. Their dreams are usually recounted as being brief, featuring few characters and simple plotlines. Research has suggested that the relationship they have with their dreams is more one of a passive observer than someone actively expressing agency. Animals play a key role in children's dreams, and the setting is often at home or a place that resembles home. As children get older and embark upon school, their cognitive development increases, as does their socialization; all of this is mirrored in their dreams, which begin to take upon more waking life concerns. With their expanded language skills, they are able to express more details of their nighttime visions. As their worlds

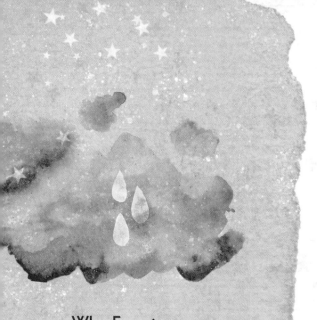

Who Experiences Nightmares?

In the general population, children have nightmares more frequently than adults. Younger children have them more often than older ones, with the incidence peaking — and then declining — at about ten years old. In adolescents, females begin to have them more often than males, a trend that continues through adulthood.

get bigger, so does the world of their dreams, with the characters that appear beginning to shift; the concentration of animals now gives way to more family members and kids of their own age.

Their dreams become more reflective of their waking life, whether related to the development of skills or the feelings they experience through interactions with family, friends, and community members. Their dreams may begin to feature multiple events strung together, rather than the isolated scenes they previously experienced. In reflecting their emotional development, action and events may be accompanied by the associated thoughts and feelings that they engender. As their imaginations continue to expand, so may the symbolic, metaphorical, and fantastical attributes of their dreams. And, as they enter school and become even more socialized, gender differences in dream content may also emerge. For example, early school-age girls report more friendly interactions than boys, who more readily note the appearance of untamed animals and aggressive interactions.

Adolescents and Teenagers

As we grow, and life concerns shift, so do our dreams. Compared to younger children, the dream settings of older kids are less reflective of waking life locales, and characters are more likely to be a compendium of numerous people. As dreams may mirror the issues that confront us, teenagers' dreams often include a focus on their changing bodies and how they feel about them, the social struggles they may have, and their growing sexual curiosity. Nightmares, while less frequently experienced than when they were younger, often include themes such as being in school, trying to escape a challenging environment, competition and sport, falling and spatial disorientation, and attacking someone or being attacked. Regarding the latter, the figure of danger in an adolescent's dream may more likely to be monsters and witches rather than actual people. Nightmares are thought to be experienced more commonly by adolescent girls than boys.

Adults

As we get older and move into early adulthood, our dream recall begins to increase. At a certain point in midlife, though, it seems to decline, whether because of more fragmented sleep, reduced interest in dreams, physiological shifts, or something else. (For ways to enhance your dream recall regardless of age, see chapter 12.) It seems that, in general, adult men dream about men more often than about women, while women dream more equally of both men and women. Nightmare prevalence is lower in adults than children, although that doesn't preclude their occurrence. Those who have had significant trauma have higher rates of post-traumatic stress disorder (PTSD), which may manifest in frequent nightmares. Compared to children, adults may be more likely to have lifestyle habits or take medications that impact their REM cycles. Adults often find themselves more interested in their dreams than when they were younger. This may reflect that in this life stage, we are inclined to be more introspective and reflective about our emotional life. Pursuing counseling or therapy also seems to have people more attuned to their dreams.

Seniors

As we enter our elder years, shifts in sleep cycles become more noticeable. The pattern changes with less time spent in stage 3 deep sleep and more in the light sleep stages 1 and 2. Studies have so far yielded conflicting results as to whether or not the percentage of time one is in REM sleep declines with advanced age. Regardless of whether sleep architecture changes in seniors shift in such a way as to reduce the total time dedicated to REM, it does seem that older people experience less REM, perhaps owing to their getting less overall sleep. As dreams reflect our waking-day concerns, their content may shift as people age, with an ensuing focus on possible themes such as scarcity, loss of resources, and their impending passing. It's been noted that older people are less likely to appear as the central figure in their own dreams. That said, it's been suggested that sexual dreams persist throughout life, and do not necessarily cease, even if a person is not as sexually active as they once were.

A Woman's Cycles and Her Dreams

Given the role that hormones play in the intricate orchestra of physiology, it's no surprise that a woman's dreams may shift throughout her life in unique ways.

DURING MENSES

Women's sleep and dreams may vary during different stages of their menstrual cycle, which makes sense, given the fluctuation of hormones that occurs. Many women find that they have more disturbances in sleep during PMS, or right after ovulation; the latter may be due to the rise in progesterone that accompanies this stage. This seems to increase basal body temperature, which may be why sleep undergoes an interference. With disrupted sleep comes shifts in their ability to recall their dreams. While it's too early to draw strong conclusions on how, and if, the menstrual cycle influences dream content, some studies have provided interesting results; PMS has been correlated with more disturbing dreams, and the pre-ovulation stage with more erotic dreams.

DURING PREGNANCY

Pregnant women report remembering more dreams than non-pregnant ones. It's unclear whether that's reflecting a hormonal shift that catalyzes a change in sleep architecture or if it's related to expectant mothers getting up more frequently in the night, which can increase their chance of waking up from a REM dream. Or perhaps it's both. Many pregnant women report dreams that are vivid and sometimes bizarre. Not surprisingly, pregnant women's dreams reflect their changing bodies, as well as the significant shift that their life is undertaking. Their dreams may mirror what they are experiencing in their lives, perhaps filled with worries or joys, allowing them to further express feelings that are arising. Images of water may be more prevalent, which may symbolize physical matters such as the buildup of amniotic fluid occurring in their body. Or it may signify more archetypal themes, such as connecting in a unitive bonding way to their child. Another commonly reported theme centers around the appearance of architectural structures; this makes sense when we think of how pregnant women experience their bodies as a container in which life is growing.

DURING MENOPAUSE

As women approach and enter menopause, many note that they are not able to sleep as well as they had previously, with shifting hormones likely to be a significant factor. There is preliminary evidence that women experiencing hot flashes are less likely to be awakened by them in the second half of the night, when more time is spent in REM sleep, than earlier. And while there is a paucity of research on how menopause and hormone replacement therapy impacts dreams, some women do report that they experience them to be different than when they were younger; this may once again mirror how dreams echo a change in life focus and concerns.

Popular Dream Themes

While dreams are individual to each person and may change through the stages of our lives, it does seem that there are some themes that show up in dreams more commonly. This makes sense, as they would reflect the shared concerns and/or inspirations that groups of people hold. As such, some may thread throughout humanity, while others may be more relevant to those of certain groups. Here are some of the most popular themes found in surveys of dreamers across cultures:

- Falling, or being on the verge of falling

- Being unprepared for a task, or trying it repeatedly

- The appearance of someone who's died

- Being chased

- Sexual experiences

- Arriving late

- Being in school

- Work

- Teeth falling out

CHAPTER SEVEN

THE ARRAY OF DREAMS

Throughout history, scholars who studied dreams have created classification systems to represent the different types that they witnessed. Reviewing these is fascinating, as it clearly reflects how our understanding of and relationship to dreams has shifted throughout time and across cultures. For example, the fifth-century scholar Macrobius put forth a five-fold division of dreams in his *Commentary on the Dream of Scipio*. His classification system held sway for quite a while, including throughout the subsequent medieval period. It included three types of predictive dreams: visio (prophetic dreams that come true), oraculum (dreams that reveal the future), and somnium (enigmatic dreams that require interpretation to discern their meaning). It also included two types of non-predictive dreams: visum (which feature the visitation of apparitions) and insomnium (nightmares, thought to be catalyzed by either physical or mental stress). Although we currently don't have a formal categorization system that everyone uses, what follows is a general sketch of the types of dreams that many people have, and the way that they are generally classified today. Given the significant role that three of these — nightmares, lucid dreams, and somatic dreams — play in the lives of many individuals, each of these will also be highlighted in more detail in subsequent chapters.

Recurring Dreams

As their name implies, these are ones that feature the same, or a very similar, situation repeating itself across numerous dreams. Recurring dreams may occur in a concentrated time period. Or, for some people, these dreams repeat throughout extended periods of their lives, with some finding themselves having dreams similar to the ones that they had when they were children. Recurring dreams are pretty common, with a majority of adults surveyed reporting that they've had them. Often, but not always, recurring dreams have negative or unpleasant tones or themes. For some people, they may be so upsetting that they are experienced as nightmares that periodically or regularly occur. It would seem that a recurring dream may be a clarion call to something toward which our psyche wants us to pay attention. They may reflect something unresolved that's calling for healing.

That said, there are different schools of thought as to why we may have them. For example, from a Jungian perspective, these dreams may reflect the cast-off parts of ourselves that are trying to gain our attention, so that we can integrate them and feel more unified. The Threat Stimulation Theory proposed by neuroscientist Antti Revonsuo suggests that these dreams give us the repeated opportunity to rehearse and refine the ways that we would face and overcome obstacles in waking life. All the while, those who suffer from PTSD may have recurring dreams in which they may continually relive their traumatic experience while they are sleeping.

Telepathic Dreams

Telepathic dreams are similar to precognitive dreams (see next page) in that both are considered to be parapsychological phenomena not able to be currently explained by science. And yet, they differ from each other. A telepathic dream is one in which a person is able to psychically transmit information to another, which then appears in that person's dreams. Sigmund Freud actually gave a nod to the idea in his paper "Dreams and Telepathy," although he supposedly never actually acknowledged belief in the idea. There are numerous anecdotal and clinical accounts of its occurrence. There's also a famous pilot study that took place at a 1971 Grateful Dead concert in Port Chester, New York. Thousands of attendees were invited to "send" thoughts of randomly selected images that were projected on a screen at the concert to a skilled dreamer miles away. Upon awakening, the dreamer reported seeing oneiric images that actually had an impressive correspondence with the art that was mentally projected by the concertgoers.

Telepathic dreams were the focus of ten years of study by esteemed dream researchers Montague Ullman, MD, and Stanley Krippner, PhD, at the Maimonides Medical Center in Brooklyn, New York. Beginning in the early 1960s, they conducted numerous research studies, eventually publishing seven articles in medical journals. While some of their participants did exhibit these paranormal dreams, given that — as they noted — it's hard to determine such a phenomenon through the scientific method, their findings weren't fully conclusive, and were difficult to replicate. One of the interesting discoveries that emerged from their research was the existence of an environmental variable that seemed to affect outcomes; telepathic dreams were found to be more frequent at times when there was less sunspot activity and fewer electrical storms.

Precognitive Dreams

This is the type of dream in which you envision an event that has yet to occur, but which eventually does so in the future. It focuses upon a happening that you had no other way of knowing about, except through your oneiric visions. Some people consider themselves to be able to foretell the future in their dreams, while others may not consider their dreams to be precognitive until after an event they dreamed about manifests. Precognitive dreams may be more commonplace than many would believe. Surveys have suggested that about half of the general public reports that they've had at least one.

Some argue against the possibility of being able to see the future, whether in waking

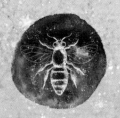

Been There, Done That...Dreamed That

Related to precognitive dreams may be the experience known as déjà rêvé, that feeling that you've already experienced something, only to realize that you did so in a dream. Some psychologists believe that déjà rêvé may explain déjà vu, that feeling that you've already lived through a current situation: you haven't necessarily been there before in waking life, but have so in a dream.

life or dreams. They note that perhaps it's just probability and coincidence. Yet, others — notably those who have had them, and those who believe in an understanding of time informed by quantum theory — swear them to be a valid phenomenon. While a nascent arena, research studies by Ullman and Krippner looked at this realm, finding that some subjects were able to dream of pictures, randomly selected by another research participant, which they had not previously before seen while awake.

While this may sound like a new-age precept, precognitive dreams are a subject that has been considered for millennia. In fact, in *On Prophesying by Dreams*, Aristotle discusses them. He doesn't necessarily support their veracity, offering that they may just be a coincidence, and yet he doesn't fully refute them either. And as we saw earlier, throughout the Middle Ages, people believed that certain dreams — such as those classified as visio or oraculum — contained insights into the future. One of the more famously cited precognitive dreams was had by Abraham Lincoln. In his dream, which the sixteenth U.S. president recounted to his wife and friends, he saw a casket being drawn by a white horse marking an assassination of a president. Thirteen days later, he was shot and killed.

Nightmares

Nightmares are bad dreams, those in which we find ourselves feeling threatened or deeply upset. They may provoke anxiety and fear, and their powerful emotional salience wakes us up. Given that we are often roused while right in the midst of one, it's no wonder that we may remember them, and that they may stay with us throughout the day (and for some people, throughout their whole life). Nightmares generally occur in the early morning hours, when we're spending more time in REM sleep.

Nightmares are most common in preschoolers, with children finding that they experience them less frequently as they enter their preteen years. Teenage girls report having them more frequently than boys their age. In children, the figures that pose a threat usually appear as monsters, ghouls, or animals, while in adults, they often take the form of other people.

It's thought that those who are more sensitive and have thinner personal boundaries have more vivid nightmares. When we are experiencing periods of helplessness in our waking life, nightmares may be more frequent. However, as upsetting as nightmares are, they are completely normal, with most everyone having them. That is, unless they happen frequently enough to cause significant distress, disrupt our sleep, and leave us with a fear of sleeping. If this is the case, they may be classified as a nightmare disorder, for which consulting a doctor may be beneficial as a means of alleviation. For much more on nightmares, see chapter 8. For information specific to children, see chapter 19.

Night Terrors

Night terrors, also known as sleep terrors, are something that many small children experience. By late adolescence, most who have had them seem to outgrow them. That said, some adults who experience traumatic events and have PTSD-informed nightmares may have night terrors. While the name may have you think that they are a type of nightmare, they actually are quite different. They occur in stage 3 SWS deep sleep, usually during the first third to half of the night. This is in contrast to nightmares, which occur during REM sleep, closer to early morning. Night terrors are sometimes accompanied by sleepwalking. No one is yet certain as to why they occur.

It can be very upsetting to experience your child having a night terror. However, rest assured that they are quite normal — estimates have it that about 40 percent of children do so. Night terrors are characterized by the sleeper sitting upright, often screaming or shouting, exhibiting a frightened expression. And while they are animated and appear to be awake, they are actually not. In fact, it's rather difficult to awaken someone from a night terror, given they are in quite a deep sleep. And it's not something that you likely want to do, as many experts suggest it's better to let a person sleep through it. Most people will have little memory of it happening the following morning. If night terrors are a challenging issue for your child, one strategy suggests waking them up a half-hour before they usually happen, so as to try to avoid their occurrence. Of course, if it's something that's of concern, speak to their pediatrician.

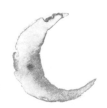

Lucid Dreams

One of the key features of a dream is that we're not actually aware that we're dreaming during them. It's only when we awaken that we become cognizant that we moved through a whole world of visions and experiences. Not so with lucid dreams. In these, while you are dreaming, you are conscious that you are actually dreaming. For some, a lucid-dream experience involves being aware you're in a dream, while for others they may also find themselves with the ability to control factors, including the environment, characters, actions, and more. While this may seem like something straight out of a modern sci-fi movie, lucid dreaming has quite ancient roots. Aristotle noted, "When one is asleep, there is something in consciousness which tells us that what presents itself is but a dream." The Greco-Roman physician Galen recommended lucid dreams as a form of therapy.

Lucid dreaming isn't as uncommon as some may think. In fact, a 2016 meta-analysis — a technique which combines data from numerous research studies — found that over 50 percent of people had noted that they had at least one lucid dream in their lifetime. Lucid dreaming is now being used by some in the psychology field to help clients who struggle with nightmares and PTSD, as well as to inspire greater creativity. For much more on lucid dreaming, see chapter 9.

Somatic Dreams

Throughout history, one of the types of dreams that was accorded with a lot of attention were those we've come to call somatic dreams. These are dreams in which we may gather awareness into the condition of our physical body, as well as connect to healing insights. Given that the prevailing paradigm of medicine doesn't emphasize a connection between the body and mind, somatic dreams are not something that currently garners the attention that they did in the past. Still, throughout history, and in cultures throughout the world, turning to one's dreams for both diagnostic and therapeutic messages was quite common. It's not only a type of dream that people recognized, but one that physicians honored and encouraged; in some societies — like that of the ancient Greco-Roman civilization — their value was so heralded that they created sanctuaries where people would go to have healing sleep and dreams. (For more on these dream temples, see page 108.)

Perhaps you've had somatic dreams. These are the ones in which you realize that your dreams are carrying forth messages that either point you toward understanding the source of dis-ease in your body and/or curative approaches that you can take to enhance your well-being. Additionally, sometimes somatic dreams leave us with strong sensations in our physical bodies, perhaps as a means of drawing attention to certain areas to which we should pay attention. (For much more on somatic dreams, see chapter 10.)

Big Dreams

Sometimes our dreams feel mundane, whereas other times they feel quite interesting and fascinating. And sometimes they exceed even that; they are highly memorable, often experienced as if they contained some very significant information or powerful lessons that we, or perhaps others, need to heed. These are what are referred to as "big dreams," a term coined by Carl Jung. Big dreams are the ones that also stick with us and we can't shake. They are the ones that feature heightened visual imagery that becomes etched into our memory. They are the ones that may immediately come to mind when someone asks you about any important dreams you've had in your life. They are the ones that may be remembered as being filled with powerful archetypes, experienced as if they are really tapping us into the collective unconscious.

Big dreams may be upsetting ones, experienced as nightmares. Or they may be joyous and revelatory ones. Cultures throughout time speak of big dreams, those that have shifted the course of people, groups, and history. Some believe that big dreams extend beyond those that have personal significance to us as individuals, to those that are envoys of insights and wisdom for the community. They connect us to something bigger, and have us feel as if we're a part of something larger than just ourselves.

Hypnagogia and Hypnopompia

You know those flashes of imagery that burst forth in your mind's eye when you're lying in bed ready to go to sleep? They have a name. Known as hypnagogia (from the Greek *hypnos* for "sleep" and *agogeus* for "leader"), these dreamlike visions, which occur in that liminal state as you drift off to slumber, often feel somewhat hallucinatory. Different than in regular dreams, in which we may find ourselves actively playing a role, in hypnagogia, we have a sense that we are more like observers than participants. Hypnagogic images tend to flicker and have a kaleidoscopic quality, and the sequence of their appearance seems to lack structural coherence.

While they may feel trippy, they are quite normal and experienced by a majority of people. (That said, if they cause you anxiety, talk to a health-care practitioner.) As striking as they are, we often can't remember them upon awakening, and only recall them if we interrupt them while they are occurring to write them down. One of the most famous proponents of hypnagogia was Salvador Dalí, who used these visions for artistic inspiration. Calling his technique "slumber with a key," he would sit in a chair with a key nestled in his closed palm and allow himself to nod off to sleep. When he did, and his muscles relaxed, the key would drop upon a plate he placed below his hand. The resulting clanging noise would wake him up, upon which time he reflected back upon the hypnagogic images that he just had, and used them as creative fodder.

Akin to hypnagogia is a phenomenon known as hypnopompia. Rather than occur between waking and sleeping, the hypnopompic state occurs between sleeping and waking. Like in hypnagogia, one may have visions that seem strange and extraordinary (hence why they are often referred to as "hallucinations"). It is sometimes accompanied by sleep paralysis, wherein you may perceive you are awake and yet your body is unable to move. Hypnopompic states seem to be less frequently experienced than hypnagogic ones.

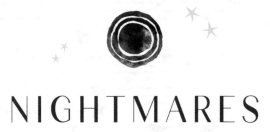

CHAPTER EIGHT

NIGHTMARES

While they are a type of dream, owing to the upset that they invoke, nightmares are anything but dreamy. And, unfortunately, they are anything but uncommon. It's thought that upward of 80 percent of people have experienced a nightmare in their lives, with estimates suggesting that about 5 percent experience them weekly. As discomforting as nightmares are, their frequency does bely something that may give you comfort: as unsettling as they may be, they are a totally normal experience. You're in good company if you have bad dreams here and there; there is nothing actually wrong with having them, besides the obvious upset that they cause.

That said, for some people, nightmares occur so regularly and with such intensity that they impinge upon their quality of life, as well as their ability to consistently get adequate sleep. In this case, one may be experiencing what's known as nightmare disorder (also referred to as anxiety dream disorder), a condition codified in the psychological guidebook, the *Diagnostic and Statistical Manual of Mental Disorders (DSM-5)*. It's estimated that about 4 percent of adults, and a greater number of children, have such powerful recurrent nightmares as to have a significant negative impact upon their well-being (whether because of ensuing emotional upset or fear of sleep). Nightmare disorder could arise in conjunction with post-traumatic stress disorder (PTSD), anxiety, depression, or other psychological conditions, or could be an outcome of an acute period of stress. Those who suffer from nightmare disorder are encouraged to seek professional assistance.

One only has to think about our everyday language to further appreciate how nightmares are an experience to which we can all relate. After all, the definition for the word is not limited to upsetting dreams — rather, it's also used to describe things that occur in our waking life. Whether employed as a noun or an adjective, the term *nightmare* describes situations or people that pose an unpleasant prospect, are difficult to deal with, or bring us fright.

Defining Nightmares

What, actually, is a nightmare? Well, if you ask medical researchers, you'll mostly find some overlap in description, but not necessarily full agreement on the nuances of how to categorically define these events. This could be the reason that among the many studies done to understand their prevalence and etiology, inconsistencies remain. Researchers aside, though, there is a general agreement that nightmares are dreams that are so upsetting and frightening that they wake us up out of sleep. Our nightmares may be filled with situations that we perceive to threaten our very survival, whether that's physically or psychologically; in our dream, we may find ourselves experiencing an assault on our physical security or our self-esteem. Sometimes they are so disconcerting that we can't seem to shake them, with their residue wafting into all corners of our waking consciousness. Years or decades later, many people still remember their first childhood nightmare.

However, not every bad dream is a nightmare. Sometimes we have dreams that contain upsetting situations or yield disturbing feelings, but they don't cause the

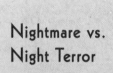

Nightmare vs. Night Terror

Nightmares are quite different than a phenomenon known as night terrors. The former occur during later episodes of REM sleep, wake you up, and are readily remembered. Meanwhile, night terrors occur during NREM sleep, generally within the first 2 hours of sleep onset, and are experienced more frequently by children than adults. In general, we remember our nightmares and yet hardly ever recall the terrifying oneiric subject matter of night terrors when we awaken. For more on night terrors and children, see page 80.

disquietude that a nightmare can. We may have plenty of bad dreams that are striking, but not stirring enough to awaken us; therefore, we recall some of what occurred, but generally not as much as the nightmares that shake us out of sleep. Nightmares, like most other vivid dreams and those with a detailed narrative structure, generally occur during the REM sleep cycle. As discussed on page 67, the length of REM cycles increases as sleep progresses through the night. As such, it seems more common to have a nightmare in the early morning hours rather than soon after you fall asleep.

THE SPIRIT OF THE NIGHTMARE

There are numerous viewpoints on what may inspire nightmares. Before we consider these, though, let's explore a mythic perspective that wove itself throughout numerous cultures, as it can help us to understand not only how people have grappled with nightmares throughout time but also from where the word itself is derived.

Mare is an old English word that denotes a creature that torments or drains the vitality of sleepers. Hence, nightmares reflect the visitation of these evil spirits in the night, during the time of slumber. Mare — also known as *mara, mart, mahrt, moroi,* or *alp* — has appeared in numerous cultural legends, including those of Germany, Croatia, and Russia, as well as Scandinavian and Slavic countries. While each spirit has its own associated myth, in general, a mare would enter into a bedroom in the evening, sit upon a sleeper's chest, and usher in bad dreams.

Legend had it that there were ways to protect against these mythical spirits and the nightmares that they catalyzed. One such strategy included preventing them from entering the room by tightly closing the doors and windows, while also obstructing all the keyholes. To initiate a detour so that they wouldn't find their way to the dreamer, shoes were left by the bedside with their toes facing the door, in the hopes that the mares would reroute themselves through the holes in which the laces were threaded. Other nightmare-prevention action plans included positioning a broom in the bedroom upside down and placing either a bundle of hay or a sharp object in one's bed. Some people would also resort to this more radical mare-dispelling custom: after urinating in a clean bottle and leaving it in the Sun for three days, they would take it to a stream and throw it backward over their head into the water. Customs that seem more aligned to strategies we may employ today to ward off disturbing dreams include sleeping in a different position and saying a prayer.

Why Do We Have Nightmares?

Mares aside, much research and inquiry has focused upon nightmares, investigating how and why they may arise, and how to address them. For some, the etiology of a nightmare may be psychological, while for others, it's a physiological factor that brings them on. What follows are a variety of perspectives on what may underlie the phenomenon.

NIGHTMARES HELP WITH EMOTIONAL PROCESSING

Many feel that through our dreams, we have the opportunity to process daytime experiences and feelings, especially those that we may not have had the inclination to digest and absorb when they occurred. Given that our lives may contain situations that are unsettling, inspire fright, feel threatening, or catalyze a host of other disconcerting emotions, it would make sense that our dreams may sometimes be upsetting, enough so to shake us up and wake us up. Nightmares may also clue us in to the unresolved psychological conflicts that we carry within.

As it turns out, those who are more sensitive, emotionally reactive, and have thinner personal boundaries are more apt to have nightmares. And of course, when we are going through acute periods of situational anxiety, stress, or grief, we may find ourselves having nightmares more frequently as we work through all the feelings in which we are swirling.

Some believe that going through the emotions stirred by an occasional nightmare can be healing, as this may give us an opportunity for processing and expression, rather than avoidance or repression. For those who believe in the prescient potential of dreams, a nightmare could also serve to alert us to an upcoming challenge. And for those who ascribe to the Threat Simulation Theory, a nightmare may be a playscape through which we rehearse actions that we can use in waking life to counter fight-or-flight situations that engender threats to our security.

NIGHTMARES CONNECT US TO THE SHADOW

Nightmares not only wake us up out of sleep, but they can also awaken us to what we may be hiding from our conscious minds. From the perspective of Carl Jung and those who practice Jungian psychology, to understand nightmares — and the route to healing that they may be revealing — we need to understand something called the shadow. The shadow is the part of ourselves that we keep in the dark, the aspects of our personality that we may deem inappropriate, hard to accept, or with which we don't readily identify. It embodies our repressed thoughts and feelings, those that we've disowned, likely due to societal conditioning. Within our shadow may reside emotions that mirror fear, shame, guilt, desire, jealousy, and unworthiness. These feelings may seem so Herculean to carry that we tamp them down and hide them away.

From a Jungian perspective, this then may constitute some of the underpinnings of nightmares: the shadow, crying out to be seen and heard, finds its outlet through dreams. And as it does, it awakens us as it rattles the cage of our emotional equipoise. The dark or gray tone inherent in nightmares reflects the shadow's overtures. In trying to get our attention, it may show up as our being chased, whether by frightening animals, demons, people, or the like. Or it may just appear emblazoned in anything that we find triggering and that blatantly catalyzes fear. And yet, by embracing these shadow elements, we encounter healing and the process of individuation that Jung so prized. Jungians assert that this can allow us to move toward holism, marrying the light and dark aspects of ourselves, weaving all the pieces of our psyche into more of a seamless tapestry. And while this perspective may not necessarily fully take away the sting that we feel when awakening from a nightmare, if we look at disturbing dreams from this orientation, we may be able to more fully appreciate the treasures of insights and healing that they offer.

It's important to remember that there is both a collective, as well as a personal, shadow. Given that some of our dreams seem to connect us directly to expressions of an archetypal nature (those that Jung called big dreams), some of our nightmares may be conduits for understanding what it is that we are together avoiding and collectively disowning. As such, some of our nightmares may be less related to personal issues and more connected to what we perceive society as a whole is repressing, whether that be despair, guilt, disempowerment, or some other form of suffering.

NIGHTMARES AS AN EXPRESSION OF EXPERIENCED TRAUMA

Those who have suffered a traumatic event often experience recurrent nightmares, which involve reminders of the episode from a physical and/or emotional perspective. In fact, having nightmares in which a traumatic event is reexperienced is one of the defining diagnostic criteria for PTSD. About 8 million Americans are estimated to suffer from PTSD, and up to 80 percent of sufferers are thought to experience nightmares. As war is one of the traumatic experiences that can cause PTSD, veterans experience it with more prevalence than the general population. Concurrently, veterans are more likely to have nightmares than the general population; in one well-cited study of Vietnam War veterans, 52 percent of soldiers had nightmares, compared to 3 percent of civilians. Other studies on veterans have found that upward of 90 percent suffer from nightmares.

Traumatic nightmares are different than regular ones, often taking a more violent tone. For some, they involve repetitive dreams that feature an exact reenactment of the anguish-filled event, unfolding as it did exactly — or exceptionally close to — as when it was originally experienced. These dreams may appear like a flashback, with daytime memory seeming to intrude upon the sleeping mind. Some traumatic dreams don't necessarily include the replayed event, but may instead be a canvas for expression of the emotions that were experienced because of it, with symbolic situations expressing terror, fear, and/or survivor guilt. Traumatic dreams are not limited to occurring in REM sleep, like regular nightmares. They may also occur in NREM sleep and be experienced as night terrors. Healing from traumatic events is often reflected in nightmare resolution.

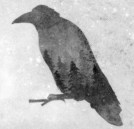

Depression and Nightmares

Not surprisingly, those with depression may have nightmares more frequently. Part of this may be explained by the finding that those with affective disorders oftentimes have challenges sleeping, which can lead to ensuing shifts in sleep architecture that contribute to the greater possibility for nightmares to occur. Not getting adequate sleep can lead to being exhausted during the day, which can impinge upon coping abilities and emotional well-being, which can exacerbate the depression-nightmare-insomnia cycle.

While some who experience PTSD-associated nightmares opt for medication, there are other behavioral approaches that have received widespread attention for their benefit, including Image Rehearsal Therapy (discussed on page 91). Lucid dreaming, which we explore in chapter 9, may also hold promise in helping people release the hold that traumatic dreams may have.

PHYSIOLOGICAL CAUSES OF NIGHTMARES

For some people, it may be physiological, rather than solely psychological, factors that give rise to their nightmares.

Medications

Certain medications are associated with the more frequent reporting of nightmares. These include antidepressants belonging to the SSRI (selective serotonin-reuptake inhibitor) category, the withdrawal from which has been associated with increased nightmares by some people. Other medications that may have similar effects include certain beta-blockers, high-blood-pressure medications, and L-dopa, the latter which is commonly used for Parkinson's disease. If you have frequent nightmares and just started taking a new medication, talk to your doctor or pharmacist to see whether bad dreams are a side effect of your prescription.

Sleep Patterns

Research studies have noted that those who have insomnia may be more likely to have frequent nightmares. Unfortunately, this can become a self-perpetuating cycle, as nightmares can lead to insomnia, owing to fear of going to sleep. This can cause sleep deprivation, which reduces resiliency and increases stress, which can then lead to more nightmares. If you notice an insomnia-nightmare connection, see chapter 2 for tips that may help you sleep better. In addition to bad dreams being more prevalent in those who don't get adequate sleep, researchers also suggest that long sleepers (those who sleep more than 9 hours a night consistently) also have more nightmares.

Other Causes

Because it shifts sleep architecture, triggering a greater concentration of REM during later cycles of sleep, heightened alcohol use has been found to be associated with nightmare occurrences in some people. Additionally, alcohol withdrawal has been found to have a similar effect. Some people with untreated sleep apnea have been found to more frequently have nightmares; using a continuous positive airway pressure (CPAP) machine may alleviate the recurrence of disturbing dreams. In some studies, stimulants such as caffeine, cocaine, and amphetamines have been found to be associated with higher occurrence of nightmares.

Rescripting the Nightmare: Image Rehearsal Therapy

Image Rehearsal Therapy (IRT) is a behavioral-based approach to treating nightmares that has garnered recognition for its efficacy. Regardless of whether a person's disturbing dreams stem from a traumatic event, are a corollary of PTSD, accompany a psychological condition such as depression or anxiety, or are just an ordinary idiopathic nightmare, IRT may be of benefit. Developed by Barry Krakow, MD, in the 1990s, IRT was recommended by the American Academy of Sleep Medicine (AASM) as a treatment for both nightmare disorder and PTSD-associated nightmares in its 2018 position paper.

IRT is a form of cognitive behavior therapy, a psychosocial orientation that suggests that psychological conditions stem from

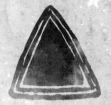

Phobetor: God of Nightmares

In Greek mythology, Phobetor was the god of nightmares. With his name meaning "fear," he was the carrier of bad dreams, often appearing as an animal or a monster in oneiric visions. He was one of the sons of Hypnos (the god of sleep) and Pasithea (the goddess of relaxation). Phobetor belonged to the Oneiri, a group of deities who personified dreams, which also included two of his brothers, Morpheus and Phantasos. While Phobetor was the name by which humans knew him, the gods called him Icelos. Many trace the mention of Phobetor to Ovid, in his opus *Metamorphoses*.

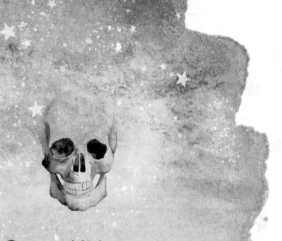

Common Nightmares

Numerous studies have been done over the years investigating common nightmare themes. One of the earliest ones dates back to the 1930s, when psychologist Husley Carson questioned over 250 people about the content of their disturbing dreams. Here's an overview of some of the most common nightmare themes uncovered in these studies:

- Physical aggression
- Interpersonal conflicts
- Failure
- Helplessness
- Health concerns
- Death
- Being late
- Falling
- Being chased
- Feeling paralyzed

faulty or unhelpful ways of thinking, as well as learned patterns of unsupportive behaviors. By addressing these thoughts and behaviors, cognitive behavior therapy has yielded promising results in treating a host of conditions. There are two main components to IRT: redefining the relationship between the dreamer and the nightmare, and a reimagining process in which the dream is rewritten.

DREAMER-NIGHTMARE RELATIONSHIP

This stage involves transforming the dreamer's association with the nightmare from one of identity to one of behavior. Instead of seeing themselves as a nightmare sufferer, they revise their perspective to see themselves as a person who has nightmares. The difference is not just semantic: there is a sense of empowerment that comes with realizing that having a nightmare is a behavior, which can be recast, rather than an aspect of identity, which is more fixed than mutable.

REIMAGINING THE DREAM

In this stage, what's first emphasized is the power of imagery, recognizing your capacity to invent stories and create new narratives, and your ability to see them visually in your mind's eye. From there, you then follow these steps:

1 Thinking of a recurrent nightmare you have, you imagine a new story arc that it can take that doesn't include the upsetting or agonizing aspects. You come up with an alternative scenario, rewriting the dream's plot, whether it be the outcome or a feature that you find triggering. Some practitioners have you write out both the original and the reimagined dreams, while others only suggest scribing the new dream, so as to avoid further emphasizing your connection to any traumatic elements in the original one.

2 Throughout the day, you allocate your attention to your reimagined dream.

3 Before bed, you replay the rewritten dream in your mind, telling yourself in a confident and encouraging way that this is the dream that you will have.

Doing the practice requires a minimal time commitment (about 15 to 20 minutes per day). And, as simple as it sounds, IRT is quite powerful. Research and clinical experiences have found that nightmare-reduction benefits may occur within weeks, and even after the practice is discontinued, benefits may still be present. IRT can be done with trained practitioners in an individual- or group-counseling setting. For those who may not want or require professional support, self-help resources like Krakow's *Turning Nightmares into Dreams*

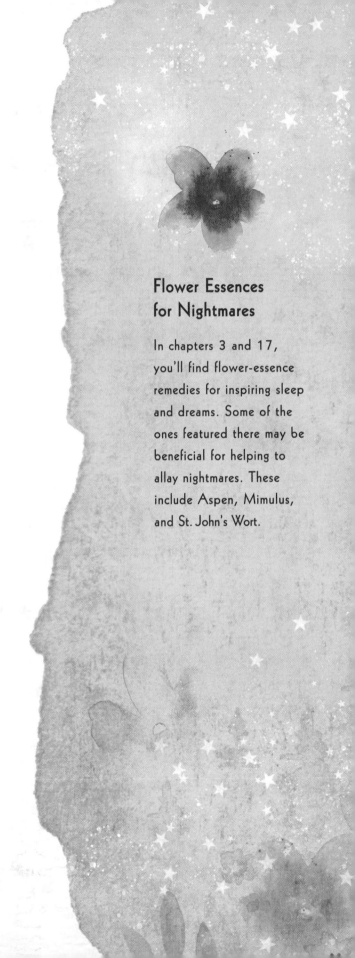

Flower Essences for Nightmares

In chapters 3 and 17, you'll find flower-essence remedies for inspiring sleep and dreams. Some of the ones featured there may be beneficial for helping to allay nightmares. These include Aspen, Mimulus, and St. John's Wort.

Self-Compassion as Treatment

Researchers have suggested that those who maintain a negative attitude toward themselves may be more inclined to experience nightmares. Given this, showering ourselves with love and forgiveness may offer yet another benefit to our well-being: being a practice that helps us counter having disturbing dreams. Here are some ways to weave more self-compassion into your life:

94

- Remember that there is no such thing as perfection.

- If something feels challenging, tell yourself that you're doing the best you possibly can.

- Every day, undertake one random act of kindness on someone else's behalf, and one on your own.

- Each evening, write in your journal at least one thing for which you are grateful.

- If you have a tendency to blame yourself for things that aren't even your responsibility, try Pine flower essence (see page 47 for more on flower essences).

book are also available. A treatment program called Examining Exposure, Relaxation, and Rescription Therapy (EERT) also features a dream reimagining component. First developed by Joanne Davis, PhD, EERT also contains a sleep-hygiene component, as well as teaches relaxation skills, including progressive muscle relaxation.

The Power of Rituals

Rituals give us grounding and have us feel that we can exact action at the behest of an intended outcome. Traditions have held that certain rituals could help to mitigate the impact of bad dreams. In Mesopotamia, they would tell their nightmares to pieces of clay and then throw them in the river to try to dispel the bad dream. The ancient Greeks would share their nightmares with the Sun, believing that its light was a spell-breaker and would cast away the darkness. However, the power of rituals to help counter nightmares may not be solely found in lore of previous times. In fact, recent studies have noted that performing rituals before experiencing a situation anticipated to be stressful can help reduce anxiety. So, if you worry about having a nightmare, doing a pre-sleep

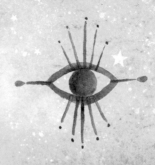

Other Therapies That Take Aim at Nightmare Disorder

In its 2018 position paper, the American Academy of Sleep Medicine shared a variety of treatments that may be beneficial for nightmare disorder. Many of these were behavioral approaches, which is good news for those who want to avoid using pharmaceutical medications. In addition to IRT already discussed, among the other therapies featured were hypnosis, lucid-dreaming therapy, and progressive deep muscle relaxation. Eye movement desensitization and reprocessing (commonly known as EMDR) is also one of the treatments that they gave a nod to when it comes to potentially treating PTSD-associated nightmares.

ritual may help to calm and center you. This may not only help you to get to sleep more readily, but provide your mind with less anxious fodder that it can translate into a bad dream.

There are many practices shared throughout the book that can help inspire relaxation, which may have the additional benefit of warding off nightmares. For example, in chapter 2 you can learn about the pacifying potency of meditation, breathwork, progressive muscle relaxation, and autogenic training.

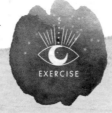

EXERCISE

The Power of Intention Setting

Another ritual that may help assuage nightmares is doing a modified version of dream incubation (a technique discussed in chapter 11). Instead of doing this practice with a particular problem-solving aim in mind, you simply focus your intention on having a pleasant dream. Before going to sleep, give a short and sweet instruction to your psyche, something to the extent of "Dream, please provide me with insights of awareness in a gentle way" or "Dream, please be filled with pleasant experiences." It may seem simple, yet intention setting can be a powerful transformative agent.

CHAPTER NINE

LUCID DREAMS

A unique feature of dreams is that we generally don't realize that they are occurring until they no longer are. As we dream when we sleep, it seems that we're often asleep during our dreams, needing to awaken to wake up to the recognition of the oneiric journey that we just experienced. But not always. It's possible to have a dream in which while it's occurring, we're able to recognize that we're actually dreaming. We're sleeping, yet not asleep to the fact we're presently dreaming. We become an awakened witness to our oneiric visions, with a cognitive cogency that perceives what is occurring. Realizing that we're in a dream, we may then choose to transform ourselves from a passive character to an active agent who can knowingly traverse dream landscapes and encounters. We can give shape to our experience, whether that means choosing to fly, transform the monsters who haunt our nightmares into allies, work through creative problems without the usual confines of Cartesian limitations, or the like.

This phenomenon is called lucid dreaming. And while for those who have never experienced it, it may sound like a plotline for a sci-fi movie (*Inception*, anyone?), it's actually something that is relatively common. In fact, it's been noted that 55 percent of people have experienced at least one lucid dream in their lifetime, with just shy of one-quarter claiming to have a lucid dream at least once a month. For those who have lucid dreams, it seems that it's an experience that begins spontaneously in adolescence.

Lucid Explorations

Lucid dreaming is considered a hybrid state of consciousness — you're in REM sleep, although not passively dreaming, and yet you're not awake, either. In this space where there's a weaving together of different levels of consciousness, you can be an oneironaut,

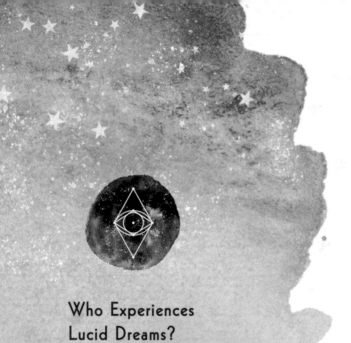

Who Experiences Lucid Dreams?

Lucid dreaming has been found to be more commonplace in those who have certain personality traits — such as openness to experience, thin boundaries, and high imaginative function — similar qualities to those who have high dream recall (as discussed on page 134). Additionally, the ability to maintain concentration and exhibit mindfulness may be helpful in lucid dreaming, reflecting studies that have shown that long-term meditators are more likely than non-meditators to be lucid dreamers.

able to explore a host of things that you may not otherwise readily be able to. After all, as you realize that dreams don't have the stability and fixity with which you had associated them, they become a canvas upon which you can more freely be an auteur. Without defenses and presuppositions both about yourself and what reality is, you can deconstruct limiting beliefs and viewpoints. You can fulfill wishes, rehearse behaviors, have adventures, and enjoy heightened sensations. You can practice skills, refine athletic moves, and learn to better understand yourself.

Lucid dreaming can be a source of spiritual understanding, an avenue to further perceive the extended nature of reality. Without your waking life defenses, you may also be more open to seeing and embracing your shadow, the oft-denied facets of ourselves to which we don't readily admit. Some have even noted that they have been able to heal illnesses through being in a lucid-dreaming state. Additionally, it's possible to rescript nightmares, which can lead to their abatement, a possible benefit reflected in the American Academy of Sleep Medicine's 2018 position paper that included lucid dreaming as a potential treatment for nightmare disorder.

THE LUCID-DREAMING BRAIN

How can it be that we're in this liminal state, with an awareness
that approaches waking consciousness while we're asleep, being in a
dream while knowing we are in a dream? Research and brain-imaging
studies may hold some clues. As we discussed in chapter 5, our brain
activity shifts when we are sleeping. One of the hallmarks of a sleeping and dreaming
brain is that one of its areas, known as the prefrontal cortex (PFC), is more dormant than
when we are awake. As the PFC is responsible for executive function — including rational
judgment, self-consciousness, and working memories — usually when we're dreaming, we
do so without an editor, judge, or witness, and without self-awareness.

However, when one is lucid dreaming, their brain looks different. EEGs taken during the
REM-sleep state of those lucid dreaming show their brains don't behave like they do in
normal dreaming. There's more electrical activity happening, reflective of a different level
of functioning than usual. This may be why during lucid dreaming people experience
metacognition and the subsequent ability to reflect upon their mental state, able to
participate in more thought monitoring than during regular dreaming. In addition to
knowing that one is dreaming, there's a greater ability to remember episodes of waking
life and volitionally control one's actions. While the PFC is more activated than it is
during regular REM dreaming, it's still more tamped down than when we are awake.
Hence, why lucid dreaming is described as a somewhat hybrid state.

A BRIEF HISTORY

Before we explore techniques that lucid dreamers use to have awareness-filled dreams, let's
look to see how our knowledge of conscious dreaming's potentiality has evolved. Lucid
dreaming galvanized attention in the 1980s, thanks to the pathfinding work of Stephen
LaBerge, PhD. A vanguard in the field, LaBerge focused his post-graduate research in
psychophysiology on the subject while studying at Stanford University. This work and his
subsequent research endeavors led to his developing a multitude of methods that are still
considered foundational for those who follow this practice. Since this time, lucid dreaming
has become a focus of study for scientists around the world, with scores of research studies
on the subject published in peer-reviewed medical journals.

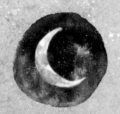

Conscious Dreaming

While lucid dreaming appears to be a modern-day pursuit, the acknowledgment that states of consciousness are not as demarcated as is often perceived is at the root of many spiritual traditions. These are the ones known for reverentially weaving a tapestry between the waking and dreaming states. Shamanic healers journey in dreams for healing insights. And in Tibetan dream yoga, you explore the nature of mind through maintaining awareness in the dreaming state to be able to experience a wider breadth of spiritual understanding.

However, it was 120 years prior to LaBerge's establishment of the groundbreaking Lucidity Institute that the pioneering tome *Dreams and How to Guide Them* was published. This initially anonymously penned book was later recognized to be authored by the French scholar Marquis D'Hervey de Saint-Denys. The treatise was based upon twenty years of research and examination of lucid dreaming by Saint-Denys, who many regard as the modern-day father of lucid dreaming. The possibility that one may have awareness in a dream was not something that was actually siloed from the psychological field. In fact, Sigmund Freud gave it a nod, noting "there are people who are quite clearly aware during the night that they are asleep and dreaming and who thus seem to possess the faculty of consciously directing their dreams" in a footnote in the 1909 second edition of his classic *The Interpretation of Dreams*. Yet, it wasn't until 1913 that the term *lucid dreaming* itself was forged. The originator of the phrase was Frederick van Eeden, a psychiatrist and the author of *A Study of Dreams*. He defined the experience as not only being able to have an awareness within your dreams, but also one in which "the sleeper remembers day life and his own condition, reaches a state of perfect awareness, and is able to direct his attention, and to attempt different acts of free volition."

Lucid-Dreaming Tools and Techniques

As we explore in chapter 12, research suggests that if you have confidence that you'll remember your dreams and you make an intention to do so, you will more likely recall them in the morning. Similar principles seem to apply with lucid dreaming. You can sow the field of conscious-dreaming potential, priming the pump, if you will, by just wanting to do so and telling yourself that it is possible.

From there, lucid dreamers use a variety of different techniques to inspire lucidity in their oneiric journeys. Different people find that certain lucid-dreaming techniques work better for them than others; therefore, experimenting with different ones may help people discover those that best align with them. While providing detailed instruction and guidance about how to lucid dream is outside the scope of this book, what follows are some of the more popular approaches that people use. (For more in-depth resources on lucid dreaming, see page 222.)

MNEMONICALLY INDUCED LUCID DREAM (MILD)

This is one of the classic methods created by LaBerge for inducing lucid dreams. The MILD method can be done when you're first going to sleep or in the middle of the night, coupling it with the Wake Back to Bed technique on the next page.

During the day, choose a dream that you recently had in which you did not experience lucidity. Run through the dream in your mind several times, looking to see if you can find any dream signs that reside within. Once you do, work on rescripting the dream, seeing yourself recognizing these as signals that you were actually dreaming. And then imagine a different path that the dream would take if you had that level of awareness. Reflect on this rescripted dream numerous times daily.

Then, when you're in bed and ready to sleep, create a lucidity affirmation in which you tell yourself that the next time you're in a dream, you will know that you are. This is a bit like dream incubation, where your conscious mind is encouraging your dreaming mind to have a certain level of awareness.

Finally, as you continue to feel lulled to sleep, go back over your rescripted dream, seeing it again and again in your mind's eye. The experience of reflecting upon being lucid, as well as having your mind be playing out a dream in the liminal state before you sink into sleep, helps to prime the psyche to have proximity to the experience of lucidity.

WAKE BACK TO BED

Another practice that lucid dreamers use involves sleep interruption, and is usually referred to as Wake Back to Bed. Given that REM sleep occurs about every 90 minutes for the average person, and the further into sleep we are, the longer the REM periods last, dreamers set their alarm clocks about 5 hours or so after going to sleep. This enhances their chance of waking up in an extended REM period. They then try to stay awake for a while, reflecting upon the dream experiences they just had; for many, doing so helps them slip right back into a lucid-rich REM dream period once they fall back to sleep.

WAKE-INITIATED LUCID DREAMING (WILD)

Hand in hand with Wake Back to Bed is Wake-Initiated Lucid Dreaming (WILD). It's the experience of moving from waking to dreaming with awareness that you're going to shift right into a dream (and, therefore, be having lucidity). As you're doing so, you're reminding yourself to notice such things as hypnagogic imagery, heavy feelings in the body, or other sensations that fill the liminal space between sleeping and dreaming. This is thought to help you slip with awareness right into a lucid dream, all the while reminding yourself that you will remember you are dreaming.

DREAM MASKS

There are numerous masks available that people use to trigger awareness that they are dreaming, an invention pioneered by LaBerge. Worn during sleep, the mask recognizes — through detecting eye movement — when you are in REM sleep. As it does, a light pulses on and off that you can sense through your eyelids. Since you would have previously made the association that the appearance of fluctuating light is a dream sign, it can trigger a moment of lucidity.

GALANTAMINE SUPPLEMENTS

An alkaloid substance known to increase acetylcholine and enhance memory, galantamine in its over-the-counter supplement form is often used for its dream-enhancing properties. (In its prescription form, it's been approved by the U.S. Food and Drug Administration for the treatment of Alzheimer's disease.) As it intensifies REM sleep, it's one of the premier compounds currently used by lucid dreamers to enhance lucidity, with research suggesting that it increases the frequency of these types of oneiric experiences. Before considering using galantamine, check with your health-care practitioner or pharmacist to ensure that it won't have a negative interaction with any current medications that you are taking or health conditions you have.

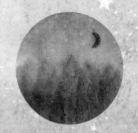

Staying Lucid

Lucid dreamers have numerous techniques they use to keep themselves in a lucid dream. Given that strong emotions often push us out of sleep, and the experience of being lucid may be quite enthralling, they remind themselves to stay calm and centered while dreaming. Some also encourage themselves to spin their dream bodies, as that seems to postpone awakenings. Another often-used trick is that they instruct their dreaming body to rub their hands together. Focusing upon this sensation is thought to help tune out sensations in the waking world that could help to sway one's dreaming attention.

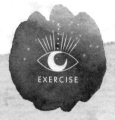

Inducing Awareness

One of the first steps in gaining awareness that you are conscious in a dream is to train yourself to make assessments of the different states of consciousness you are in at any time. Most of us live our lives just assuming we are awake, taking it for granted. Knowing how we know we're awake, lucid-dream experts note, is key to knowing how to know that we're dreaming.

To practice inducing awareness, during different parts of the day, do what's called a reality check. It's a simple technique; just ask yourself, "Am I dreaming?" Doing so enables you to identify what the signs are that have you know that you are actually awake, which can help you then realize the unique signs that reveal when you are in a dream. It also gets you into the habit of asking this question, so that you can more readily inquire about this when you are actually dreaming.

The other benefit of doing this practice is that it enhances our sense of mindfulness during our waking moments. After all, when we ask ourselves "Am I dreaming?," our attention becomes focused and we perceive the world with more clarity. This can help us not only hone our awareness when it comes to discovering lucidity in our dream life, but in our waking life as well.

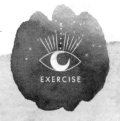

Looking for Dream Signs

One way to assess whether you are dreaming is to identify what are known as dream signs. These are the signals that indicate you are actually in a dream, as they are events that either likely or definitely cannot occur in waking reality, characteristics that only occur in the dream state.

A good place to start in finding your dream signs is to go through your dream journal (see chapter 14), reviewing it to see whether there are places, events, people, or perspectives that forge recurring roles in your dreams. Pay special attention to those that don't appear in your waking life at all or don't appear in the same pattern as they do in your dreams.

Compile a list of these dream signs, perhaps dedicating a page or so in your dream journal to them for handy reference. Before you go to sleep, review these dream signs. This way, you'll be honing your attention so that if you see them in your dream, you will be more likely to recognize that you are actually dreaming.

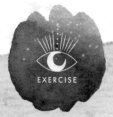

Practicing Text Reading

One of the signs that many people believe heralds that we're in a dream is the way that we experience writing. We know that when we're awake and we look at a written document it appears a certain way. And regardless of whether we turn our attention away from a page in a book, for example, once we return our focus to it, the words look and read just as they did before.

Yet, when we dream, words oftentimes morph: they can shift position, size, color, and meaning. So, if you see text in your dream, focus your attention on it, reading it a couple of times. If the text shifts in any way, that may be enough of an Aha! to trigger your awareness that you are, in fact, in a dream.

One recommended strategy to strengthen your ability to remember to do this in a dream is to practice it several times during the day. It's simple to do: just read a piece of text, turn your attention away, and then read it again. You will see that it remains static, reinforcing to you that you're awake, and not in a dream.

CHAPTER TEN

SOMATIC DREAMS

Cultures with healing traditions that honor the connection between the mind and the body perceive that certain dreams offer insights that can help us to understand and improve our well-being. In this chapter, we'll explore these types of oneiric visions, referred to as somatic dreams. We'll do so by discussing the ancient dream temples, as well as the perspectives of physicians and philosophers esteemed throughout history. We'll also look to several systems of traditional medicine in which dreams play an important role in both diagnosis and treatment. In addition, we'll explore the range of expression that somatic dreams can take, as well as recent research that may shine light on what they can reveal, and how we can turn to our dreams for healing insights.

Sanctuaries of Dream Healing

Back in times past, dreams played an integral role in the collective approach to healing for many societies. One of the most stellar examples of this was the prominence in some ancient cultures of sacred dream temples. Think of them somewhat akin to our modern-day medical spas. Those seeking relief from illness would travel to these sanctuaries and engage in prescribed rituals, in hopes of having a dream that would include healing insights.

These sanctuaries include ones found in ancient Egypt that date as far back as four thousand years ago. Many of these dream temples were dedicated to Imhotep, once chancellor to pharaoh Djoser, who was later deified as a god of medicine and healing. As part of a healing regimen offered at these sites, those looking for respite would be lulled to sleep through hypnotic suggestions; these were given by the temple priests and priestesses, who would later interpret the supplicants' dreams. The sleep-lulling prompts were thought to influence a person's ability to connect to divine healing inspiration in their sleep. The Egyptian sleep sanctuaries laid part of the foundation for what currently remains one of the better-known dream sanctuary traditions: the Asklepieia, the ancient Greco-Roman dream temples.

THE ASKLEPIEIA

If you think back to the pantheon of Greek deities, you may remember Asclepius. While many recall him as the god of medicine, what is not as well known is how dreams comprised a large role in the healing system that he forged and practiced. According to Edward Tick in *The Practice of Dream Healing*, Asclepius's father, Apollo, gave his son "prophecy and dream visitations as divine gifts." Physician-priests who followed in the traditions of Asclepius created healing temples throughout the ancient Mediterranean region that were named after him: they were collectively known as Asklepieia, with singular temples called Asclepeion. About three hundred of these ancient temples of dream healing have so far been discovered. The most famous Asclepeion dates back to the fifth century BCE and is located in Epidauros, in the northeastern area of the Peloponnese region of Greece, which is said to be Asclepius's burial site.

Those looking for healing would travel to an Asclepeion. There, they would engage in a series of purification rituals, which included dietary restrictions, ritualistic bathing, and the use of therapeutic herbs. Some of the temples featured large amphitheaters where dramatic productions would take place, meant to inspire the stirring of emotions and resultant cathartic release. This preparatory work was thought to invoke the supplicant's conscious participation in the healing process, including cultivating their faith as well as their psychological readiness.

This was all done in advance of their entering into a special chamber, known as an *abaton*. Here, they would sleep, either on the floor or on stone beds covered with animal pelts. Walking barefoot and dressed in special robes, they would be escorted to the abaton by a physician-priest, who would lead them in a final prayer before they were left in silence to sleep and receive a healing dream. Temple sleep was known as *enkoimisis*.

Once asleep, they awaited the "arrival" of Asclepius or his proxies — snakes, dogs, and roosters — in their dreams. It was said that the dream god sometimes would ask questions and then offer curative suggestions, such as herbs, medicines, foods, or rituals. Other times, spontaneous healing was said to occur through a direct encounter; this could arise from just seeing Asclepius in a dream, or having his surrogate animals appear to touch the dreamer. There are even reports of some people recounting that they were operated upon. Often, Asclepius would invite the dreamer to create art — including composing songs or skits — as a means to further their healing, owing to the perceived ability of these activities in restoring emotional balance.

Still, it wasn't always that the dream's therapeutic value was immediately obvious. It's said that sometimes Asclepius would incorporate riddles or puns into them, which needed to be deciphered. This was one of the reasons that part of the healing ritual included having the physician-priests act as interpreters, helping to discover and discern what came through in a dreamer's nighttime visions, further amplifying the healing.

And while all this may sound extraordinary, there are numerous accounts of people arriving at Asklepieia with physical and emotional maladies, only to leave these sacred healing spots replete with health. These records include not only inscriptions carved into the temple walls but also plaques and votive offerings placed as symbols of gratitude; these votives were often in the shape of body parts, inscribed with the donor's name, presumed to have been the area of healing in which they experienced relief. Reflecting upon these ancient temples gives us a historical and cultural context for the role that dreams played in ancient civilizations. It also shows us the inherent healing power that dreams may have.

Somatic Dreams: A Historical Perspective

When we view the dream temples through our current-day lens, they may seem rather odd. However, if we put them in the context of the times, it makes more sense. In ancient civilizations, part of the reverence accorded to dreams was their healing benefit, which was not just limited to the emotional realm; rather, dreams were also viewed as a means to further understand and bolster physical well-being. After all, for most of history, health was seen as unitive, with the body, mind, and spirit having an integrated relationship. If we see illnesses as having a psychospiritual component, we can further understand how dreams may be valuable in their ability to reveal insights about our physical health. Let's take a look at some esteemed figures in the history of medicine to further frame the context in which dreams were understood.

HIPPOCRATES

Hippocrates, often referred to as the father of Greek medicine, was one of the first to write about dreams and physical health, including in his work *On Dreams*. Many of the medical treatises with which he is associated include reference to the role of sleep and dreams, and the diagnostic value they hold for understanding somatic symptoms. For example, in one of his books he noted that dreams of fountains may indicate a disorder stemming from the bladder.

ARISTOTLE

Aristotle wrote three books on the subject of sleep and dreams: *On Sleep and Dreams, On Sleeping and Waking,* and *On Divination Through Sleep*. He suggested that dreams evolved as a result of sensations we had in our waking life, as well as what our minds perceived occurring in our bodies during sleep. As such, he noted that within dreams, we may be able to find information on events taking place somatically, reflecting the notion that oneiric visions can have diagnostic functions.

GALEN

Galen of Pergamon was a well-regarded physician thought to have forged the foundation of Greco-Roman medicine. The author of *On Diagnosis in Dreams*, he did some of his early medical training at an asklepeian healing temple. One of the principles that he promoted was that dreams have healing and medical diagnostic abilities. He seemed to have believed that physicians had a special capacity to make prognostications related to dreams, noting that these were superior to those made by diviners and others who interpreted oneiric visions.

AVICENNA

Ibn Sina, also known as Avicenna, was a highly regarded physician of the medieval Islamic world whose work influenced medical-school curriculum for centuries to come. He noted how images in dreams may reflect different body constitutions; for example, those with hot temperaments may dream more of the Sun while those with cold temperaments may dream of being submerged in freezing water. He asserted that dreams could also help identify imbalances in humours, the four fluids that formed the centerpiece of medical thought in ancient and medieval medicine.

Types of Somatic Dreams

Even if our current medical approach doesn't feature a consideration of dreams, that's not to say that there aren't people studying this field, nor numerous reports of dreamers who've had firsthand experience with health-related dreams. There are also many anecdotal reports of people who have had somatic dreams related to their physical health. Somatic dreams generally fall into one of four categories, including:

DIAGNOSTIC

These dreams, also called prodromal or pathognomic dreams, occur before either the onset of noticeable disease symptoms or a disease diagnosis. There are numerous accounts of people who have had dreams that contained imagery that had them wondering whether they had a health condition. While they may not have had outward symptoms reflective of a disease, and therefore remained without diagnosis from a physician, they convinced their doctor to perform the necessary tests, only to find confirmation. For some of these people, their dreams were able to save their lives; if left untreated, their illnesses may have led to health deterioration and/or death.

SYMPTOMATIC

These are dreams that a person may have after they realize that they are experiencing dis-ease or have been diagnosed with a health condition. Through these dreams, they may gain more insights into physiological shifts that have taken place in their body. These dreams may also allow for the working through of emotions that have been catalyzed owing to their condition or the impact that their symptoms have upon them.

PRESCRIPTIVE

Like in the dreams of asklepeian supplicants, many people have reported that they received oneiric insights about a pathway to take to resolve a current illness or stem the possibility of the development of one. One famous example of this comes from the account of British architect Sir Christopher Wren. Upon his taking ill, he postponed having a bloodletting treatment until the following day. The dream he had that evening included scenes of palm trees and a woman offering him some date fruits. The next morning he decided to eat some dates and subsequently found himself to be healed of his illness.

CURATIVE

There are also accounts of people being spontaneously healed in their dreams. While the imagery varies, some report that in the dream itself someone appears and says that they will help heal the sufferer and/or performs an act of healing in the dream. They then subsequently find that their symptoms have mitigated upon arising, or shortly thereafter.

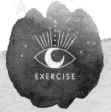

EXERCISE

Tuning in to Your Somatic Dreams

Now that you know more about these types of oneiric visions, survey your dreams to see whether you've ever had one (or several) that were somatically informed. For example, thinking back to the last time you weren't feeling well, look back in your dream journal to the dreams you had around that time. See whether there are any symbols that appeared that, in retrospect, seem like they were reflecting the experience of dis-ease. If so, keep note of them in case they appear in subsequent dreams.

You can also use the dream incubation technique to try to discover curative solutions for when you're feeling under the weather. Before going to bed, ask your dreams to reveal insights on dietary guidance and self-care practices that may help you feel better. In the morning, look to what arose in your dreams through the lens of your wellness inquiry. To learn how to practice dream incubation, see chapter 11.

Dreams in Healing Systems the World Over

Except for in psychotherapy, modern Western medicine does not generally carve out a place for dreams. That is not true, though, when it comes to traditional healing systems that offer a more holistic and body-mind-spirit paradigm, including Ayurveda and traditional Chinese medicine, as well as the integrative medical approach known as homeopathy. Dreams also play a role in the healing approaches of many traditional cultures.

AYURVEDA

Ayurvedic medicine is a classical Indian healing system. Noting that *ayur* means "life" and *veda* means "wisdom" or "knowledge," it is seen as the science of life and longevity. Ayurveda honors the connection between mind, body, and spirit. It emphasizes the healing potential of diet, lifestyle habits, and nature-based medicine. While gaining popularity in the West in recent decades, it has longstanding roots in India, with the earliest texts on Ayurveda dating back thousands of years. Ayurveda notes that the character of our dreams is influenced by the quality and quantity of the sleep we have, itself influenced by our diet and lifestyle routines. Since ancient times, dreams were used in Ayurveda to offer insights on the diagnosis or prognosis of a disease. Dreams are referred to as *svapna* and thought to reflect the interweaving of four integral components: the physical body, mind, soul, and sense organs.

One way that Ayurveda addresses health is by ensuring that a person's unique temperament is balanced. There are three constitutions, also known as doshas: these are vata, pitta, and kapha. According to Ayurveda, dreams can be used to identify a person's dosha or see whether doshic imbalances currently exist.

- Vata dreams may include flying, climbing trees, and other general movements. They feature dry and arid environments, vivid images, and scenes that conjure anxiety.

- Pitta dreams may feature fire, lightning, the Sun, and the color gold. They may include action and adventure, as well as competition and conflict.

- Kapha dreams are more placid, and feature calming scenes in which nature or water may be highlighted. Birds, clouds, or milk may be included, and attachment is often a theme.

Another vantage point through which classic Ayurveda views dreams is their ability to infer the timing of an outcome of a prognostic dream. In one of the Ayurvedic texts, the *Harita Samhita*, it's noted that if the dream took place in the first part of the night, the results were to occur in one year; in the second part, in six months; in the third part, in three months; and in the fourth part, in ten days. It was also thought that pregnant women could get a sense of the gender of their baby in their dreams. For example, if a dream featured flowers such as lotus or water lily, the baby was likely to be a boy. Alternatively, if a dream included flowers such as rose or hibiscus, the woman was likely to give birth to a girl.

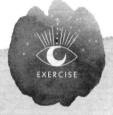

EXERCISE

Know Your Dosha

Interested in learning more about the intersection of Ayurveda and dreams? One of the first places to start is by learning which dosha (constitution) you are. While consulting with an Ayurvedic practitioner is the most thorough way to receive a dosha determination, you can also find quizzes online that will help you to understand which one you may be. Once you know your dosha, see whether your dreams accord with the qualities noted for each (see page 113). If you track your dreams over time through this angle and find that your dosha-associated themes significantly shift, it may be signaling that your body and mind are somehow out of balance. As you make adjustments in your diet and pursue practices that reduce stress, see how that may be reflected in your dreams.

TRADITIONAL CHINESE MEDICINE

Traditional Chinese Medicine (TCM), which has been practiced for thousands of years, has also gained prominence around the world in the last decades for its holistic and efficacious approach. It features body/mind practices such as acupuncture, herbal medicine, nutrition, tui na massage, qi gong, and other modalities. TCM addresses the energetic flow of the body, identifying different symptoms and emotions associated with each major organ.

Dreams are given high accord in this medical approach. They themselves are explained in a unique way; as Giovanni Maciola shares in his book *The Practice of Chinese Medicine*, dreams are due to the nighttime wanderings of the mind (known as the Ethereal Soul). During the day, the Ethereal Soul resides in the liver, while at night when it moves to the eyes, it inspires dreaming. TCM doctors usually ask about the frequency and nature of a patient's dreams in order to further assess their health status. It's thought that a healthy person should have sleep not disturbed by excessive dreams; although what excessive constitutes isn't clear, some practitioners characterize it as frequent nightmares or anxious dreams, or waking up exhausted after having many active dreams.

In the TCM classic text *The Yellow Emperor's Classic of Medicine*, it's noted that dreams are influenced by the balance of the complementary, yet opposing, forces of yin and yang. Another factor that's discussed is how dreams may reveal whether there exists an energy deficiency or excess in one of five organs (liver, heart, spleen, lung, and kidney). According to TCM, what you dream about can also be helpful for diagnosing health imbalances. Within the ancient Chinese texts, you will find many dream images and what they represent healthwise. For example, they note that if your liver is deficient in energy, your dreams may include fragrant mushrooms or forests. If it's spring and you dream of lying under a tree and are unable to get up, that may reflect liver deficiency; alternatively, dreams in which you're angry may point to liver excess. Being immersed in water, swimming after a shipwreck occurs, or overlooking an abyss are thought to reflect weak kidneys, while if one dreams of volcanic eruptions in the summertime, it may signal that the dreamer's heart is not strong. Different colors in dreams are thought to also reveal insights. Red is associated with the heart; white, the lungs; black, the kidneys; green, the liver; and yellow, the spleen.

HOMEOPATHY

Created in the late eighteenth century by the German physician Samuel Hahnemann, homeopathy is a holistic medical system that is currently practiced worldwide. Homeopathy maintains an integrative vision that takes mental and emotional well-being into consideration along with physical health. Homeopathic remedies are very dilute forms of natural substances, thought to restore health through operating on a subtle energy level.

To find the correct remedy, a homeopath will do an extensive consultation with a patient, inquiring into an array of subjects, including ascertaining details related to their medical history, lifestyle, personality traits, and dietary preferences. Additionally, they not only gather information about sleep patterns, but also ask about a patient's dreams, including how well they recall them, the tone of their dreams, and any striking recurring images. They will then take all this information and use it to find a remedy that will be a match for the person, one that may restore their client to better health. Part of the way that they do this is by turning to a book known as a repertory. Within it, they can look up the personal factors — including dream reflections — that their patient recounted to see which remedy may accord with them.

One look at *The Phoenix Repertory* by Dr. JPS Bakshi can yield insight into just how dreams are used in homeopathy to determine a person's correct treatment. Within this classic book is an entire thirty-plus-page section dedicated to dreams, featuring hundreds of different oneiric qualities and the remedy, or remedies, associated with them. For example, dreaming of a hot stove points to the remedy Apis, visions of picnicking refer to Nat Sulph, the appearance of elephants suggests Kali Mur, and being lost in the woods points to Sepia. Further underscoring how dreams can be used for therapeutic purposes, there is an array of different remedies depending upon key nightmare features. For example, nightmares occurring in the morning indicate different remedies than those that may have been dreamt before midnight, which differ from those that occur after midnight.

A nightmare dreamed by a woman after her period yields one remedy, while one dreamed in her premenstrual cycle indicates another. And if you're a person who frequently has nightmares during Full Moons, this will have your homeopath further research whether it's Nat Carb that is the right remedy for you.

MAASAI MEDICINE

The Maasai, an ethnic group who live in parts of Kenya and Tanzania, ascribe a lot of meaning to dreams, honoring them for their guidance and valuing them as a vital part of life. Morning rituals often include sharing dreams with those with whom you gather. Part of the approach that spiritual healers, known as *laiboni*, use to treat those seeking counsel is through interpreting their dreams. There are additional ways that dreams serve as founts for valuable insights: for example, according to Dr. Tanya Pergola in *Time Is Cows: Timeless Wisdom of the Maasai*, elders seeking more information about the sacred sites where they could potentially host an *orlpul* — a healing retreat — often look to their dreams to discover it.

YORÙBÁ MEDICINE

Also known as Orisha medicine, Yorùbá is a healing system popular in West Africa and the Caribbean. To help the community, traditional healers use a variety of techniques, including herbal medicine, the telling of folktales, intentional dancing, and dreams and dream interpretation. As the ancestors are thought to visit in a person's dream, Yorùbá healers receive healing wisdom from them in their oneiric visions. Additionally, the healer will not only ask their client about their recent dreams to try to further understand what may be ailing them, but they may also rely upon information that came through in their own dream for this aim. This can inform not only the diagnosis but also any helpful remedies and treatments that they may prescribe.

TIBETAN MEDICINE

Dreams have played an ongoing role in Tibetan medicine. Even before the arrival of Buddhism to Tibet in the seventh century, dream analysis maintained an integral role in medical knowledge as well as spiritual practice. Not only do physicians inquire about their patients' dreams, but they may also conjure a dream about them before their visits in hopes of attaining more insight into their prevailing condition. It's thought that dreams can be informative in all stages of a disease: before it manifests, during its process, and after it's been cured. Dream images are seen as representing symbolic snapshots of the parts of the body that may be infirmed.

Research into Health-Related Dreams

At this point, there is a dearth of scientific research into the intersectionality of dreams and health. That said, some exploration has been undertaken and has yielded fascinating results. One of the leading contributors to this realm was the Russian psychiatrist Vasily Kasatkin. Over a forty-year period, he created a database of over ten thousand dreams compiled from more than 1,200 people. Through analyzing their dreams, he found that many contained symbols that served as precursors to the development of illness; that illness-catalyzed dreams are filled with distress and are generally longer than other dreams; and that dreams can point toward the physical location of a disease. His findings are included in his book *Theory of Dreams*, which has recently been translated into English. In it, he notes, "Describe me the dream of a person and I will tell you what illness he suffers from."

Another person known for their research exploring how dreams may be related to illness is psychiatrist Robert Smith of Michigan State University. In the 1980s, he undertook two studies on the subject: "The Relationship of Dreaming and Being Ill" and "Dreams Reflect Biological Function." One of the striking findings suggested by his studies is that the severity and deterioration of a health condition is associated with themes portrayed in dreams. For example, he found that in men, it was dreams of death that correlated with the subsequent worsening of disease symptomology, while in women, it was dreams that featured themes of separation.

Another pioneer in the field is Patricia Garfield, PhD. One of the founders of the International Association for the Study of Dreams, Garfield has done a lot of exploration into the role that dreams play in health and well-being. In her book *The Healing Power of Dreams*, she recounts not only the role that dreams played in her own recovery from an injury, but also those of countless others whose oneiric visions provided them with diagnostic and therapeutic insights. In her book, she includes an amalgamation of numerous dream images and the health conditions with which they have been found to be associated.

Envisioning Your Health Through Dreams

This is not to say that every dream you have that features a certain image or scene means that you have an undiagnosed illness. Still, it may be interesting to pay close attention to your dreams to see if they offer you a compass that can further help you tune in to what you are experiencing on a somatic level. If you find yourself having a dream with a recurring theme, and you intuitively feel that it may be pointing to some underlying physiological weakness, consider discussing this with a doctor or other health-care professional. If you are under the weather, or dealing with a physical condition, remember the ability of dreams to provide us with under-the-radar wisdom. Listen in to your dreams to see if you can gather insights on how to bolster your health and well-being. Perhaps use this as a focus of your dream incubation, asking your oneiric visions to bring you awareness about curative suggestions that you could then research. (For more on incubating a dream, see chapter 11.) Additionally, some people have noted that through lucid dreaming, they are able to overcome some underlying stress associated with health conditions that they may have. If this is of interest to you, consider consulting a health-care practitioner who practices lucid-dream therapy.

119

In the West, our vision of the healing potential of dreams is mostly limited to a psychotherapeutic perspective, rather than a somatic one. However, as more and more people turn to their dreams for insights, and we continue to move toward a health paradigm that embraces mind, body, and spirit, perhaps one day doctors will not only inquire about your sleep but will also routinely ask you, "How are your dreams?"

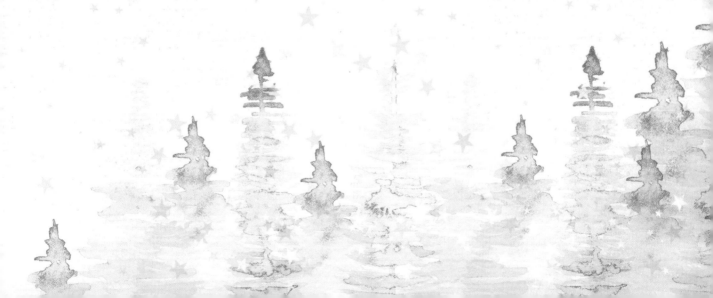

dreamwork practices

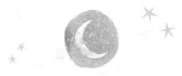

CHAPTER ELEVEN

DREAM INCUBATION

What's your go-to strategy for creative problem solving? For some, it's ringing up a friend. For others, it's talking with their therapist, while for others, it may involving twirling the quandary around in their mind again and again, hoping that a solution emerges. But did you know that there's another technique for unearthing personal and professional insights that involves actively turning to your dreams?

Known as dream incubation, this nighttime intention-setting practice involves consciously asking our dreams to bring forth awareness about a particular topic upon which we are focused. While it may sound newfangled, it's anything but. Since time immemorial, people have been consciously practicing dream incubation, which featured a host of rituals, techniques, and routines to help generate dreams that would offer them breakthroughs and healing. And while these were multi-spectrum approaches that involved pre-slumber rituals and sleeping in sacred sanctuaries, as they did in the Asklepieia discussed on page 108, they also involved trusting that the dream that they would experience would offer them solutions to problems they were facing.

Currently, in popular culture, the term *dream incubation* is defined more narrowly, as the pre-sleep practice of intentionally asking your dreams to provide you with insight on a certain topic. It can yield amazing results and is something that's been used by artists, inventors, business leaders, and others to generate answers to creative and everyday life problems. It's a technique that psychotherapists who use dreamwork teach to their clients. And it's something about which you can find published research in medical journals documenting studies that show how it can be helpful with problem solving. It's not a difficult practice that requires special skills nor one that takes a lot of time. The main

121

thing that it requires is the belief in the wisdom of your dreams, that within you resides the answers that can help you navigate your life with more clarity and awareness.

Minding Our Intentions

Dream incubation allows us another way to more deeply etch the two-way dialogue between our conscious and subconscious minds. It invokes the will of the mind to make a declaration of intent, which may be heard by the subconscious. In this practice, we are planting seeds in the garden of our psyche, envisioning the blossoming of dreams that yield knowledge and healing. We're asking our dream minds, with reverence and intention, to share with us understanding about something that isn't fully yet clear to us. We query our dreams in a deliberate manner, asking that they provide us with answers to questions or challenges we are facing, or problems we would like to solve. As you are going to sleep, you turn your conscious attention to something about which you'd like more awareness. Are you struggling with a relationship quandary? Perplexed by whether you should pursue a job opportunity you just learned of? Uncertain how to support your child in the current challenge they're facing? Whatever you're at a standstill with, the things about which you would like to have a breakthrough can be fodder for your dream-incubation practice.

Life issues are not the only realm of potentiality, however, when it comes to this practice. It can be a powerful technique to use for gaining creative breakthroughs. If you're working on a technical or an artistic project and the next steps just seem to keep alluding you, turning to your dreams may provide you the out-of-the-box thinking you need. The ideas that may come forth may be just the ones you need to catalyze your process to illuminate the next steps to take. As we explored in the Introduction, artists and inventors who were struggling with creative problems found that it was from their dreams that innovative solutions would emerge.

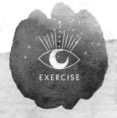

How to Do Dream Incubation

Here's an easy step-by-step guide to doing dream incubation. On first blush, it may seem rather involved, but actually it's not; it's something that you only need to spend about 10 minutes each day to do.

Step 1: Choosing Your Focus

The focus of your dream-incubation query should be something truly significant, something that really matters to you and your happiness. As the process invariably honors the sacred wisdom inherent in our dreams, the question shouldn't be about a frivolous topic. It shouldn't be something whose answer would just be interesting, but rather something whose answer would be truly meaningful and life-affirming. Research has shown that dream incubation works better when the dreamer has an emotional connection to the issue and a strong desire to find the solution. It's also been found to be more productive when the topic is something that the dreamer has been struggling with, working hard to find a solution to in their waking life, yet about which they still feel blocked. Therefore, avoid topics for which you haven't tried to yet find a resolution. It's not so much that dream incubation is a last-line strategy, but rather that there seems to be something essentially valuable about the process of already being actively steeped in the query itself that can bring forth innovative paths to resolution.

It shouldn't be difficult to come up with a topic; after all, it's likely something that's been bothering you and something about which you feel really uncertain. It can be in any realm of your life: your career, a relationship, a family dynamic, a wellness pursuit, or something else that's fully capturing your attention. It may be a situation that you know to be emotionally triggering, and yet, you're just not clear what's really underneath the feelings that are being stirred within. Or, perhaps, the subject is related to a creative project you've been working on and about which you're still finding yourself at an impasse, not sure how to move forward. Any and all of these could be great fodder for dream incubation.

As you hone in on the subject, ensure that it is something about which you truly want to know the answer, something you will act upon and for which you'll take responsibility if you do. Ask yourself whether if you had more insight on a certain subject you would be ready to follow through, or whether it is a situation that you're currently hesitant to resolve. If there's a disconnect between your interest in finding a pathway forward and your ability and/or willingness to make significant life shifts, your dreams may not provide you with the awareness you truly know you're not really ready for anyway. Or if they do, you could find that having the understanding about how to move forward but not actually doing so may end up causing dissonance. This practice should be powerful and uplifting rather than feel like it's adding more stress and discord to your life. That said, if you intuitively know that getting some insight may help motivate you to break out of a pattern, then it may be a focus that is beneficial.

Step 2: Framing the Question

Now that you know the domain of life for which you're interested in getting more insights, it's time to come up with your incubation question. Composing a well-asked question is key. The question is not only the carrier of the intention but also the scope through which you'll understand what your dream has brought forth. You don't want it to be too general or broad, yet you don't want it to be excessively narrow, either. It should be straightforward and precise, simple yet targeted. It should be an open-ended rather than a close-ended question, the latter being one that involves a Yes or No answer.

It's much better to ask about one facet of your dilemma rather than a multitude. This way, when you survey what has come through in your dream, you'll know just what it is answering. This will help reduce uncertainty as to whether what arose in the dream applies to one part of the question or another. For example, it's better to ask, "What is something that I continually avoid acknowledging about the way I interact with my partner?" rather than "What is something that I continually avoid acknowledging about the way I interact with my partner, why do I do that, and what should I do about it?" If you asked the multi-prong question you may not necessarily know which part of it the dream was answering. It will be much more straightforward and obvious with a pointed question.

Once you've come up with your initial question, sit with it for a minute or two. See how it feels, tuning in to whether or not it hits the mark for you. Give yourself flexibility to adjust it if you feel it can be more aligned. Write the question down in your journal. Remember one more thing: dreams are very visual. Therefore, see if you can frame the question in a way to allow for the answer to appear in something that is seen, rather than something that is solely heard or accessed via another of the senses.

Step 3: Asking the Question

Pose the question to yourself in a way that reflects the significance of your inquiry, sculpting it as if you were asking it of someone who held a key that you were looking for (as you, and your dreams, do). Be sincere, direct, and reverent, reflecting your commitment to want to know the answer. Ask that the answer that is revealed in your dreams be shown to you in a way that is readily understandable and recognizable.

You can say the question out loud or quietly in your mind. Let it be like a mantra, prayer, or lullaby. Focus your attention upon it as you drift off to sleep. Images may arise during the hypnagogic period — that gossamer state between awake and asleep when hallucination-like forms seem to appear. Allow those to emerge, and don't worry if in the morning you can't remember them (we usually can't). Trust that they are setting the stage for a revealing dream to occur.

Step 4: When You Awaken

First, follow the steps outlined in chapter 12 on how to awaken consciously to your dreams. Then, record your dream, using the strategies outlined in chapter 13. At first, don't try to understand the dream in the context of the question. Just write down everything you remember without interpreting it. At this point, you're not looking for the dream to fit the shape of the intentionally constructed question; you want to fully access what transpired and not restrict anything. Later on, you can then reflect upon the dream to see what insights it has revealed related to your inquiry. When's later on? It can be right after you've recorded it or anytime during the day when you're focusing upon your dreamwork.

Remember that the dream may reveal the solution directly. Or, it may be more clearly understood through the lens of symbols or images that wove through the dream. If the dream seems relevant to your focus, you may get answers that reflect an action to take. Or you may not. Rather, it may give you further insights into how you are feeling, or perhaps more awareness about the situation that wasn't previously apparent. If the dream revealed relevant information, you may want to synthesize it with your waking-life thoughts on the matter. Marrying them may yield a solution that offers greater potentiality for seeing the best step forward than either one alone.

Once you have what appears to be an answer, sit with it and see how it feels. Do you have a sense of positivity as if a cloud has lifted? Remember that you can do follow-up dream incubations. You can incubate the same question of focus again if you want further understanding, or you can reframe it based upon the new insights that already undertaken ones have yielded.

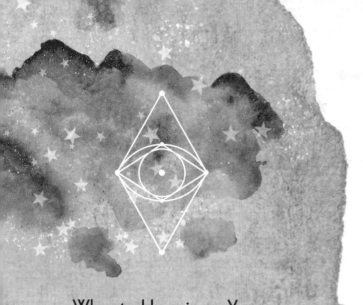

When to Hone in on Your Dream Incubation Focus

Some people like to concentrate on their dream incubation as they're winding down in bed. They survey their day and zero in on what may have emotionally triggered them or what consideration they feel they are still grappling with. Others like to begin to concentrate on their dream incubation realm beforehand. Throughout the day, they open their mind's eye to situations that feel provocative, having that direct them to discover the topic for their nighttime inquiry. Yet, others may wait until their evening relaxation time — say, while they're bathing or writing in their journal — and turn their attention then to the sphere of life that's of most interest to them to resolve.

ENCOURAGING THE INCUBATION

In addition to the question carrying the intention of your query, there are practices you can do to further encourage your dream to zero in on your realm of interest.

- Place objects in your bedroom — either on your nightstand, dream altar, or some other place visible from your bed — that reinforce your question. For example, let's say you're seeking guidance on a relationship, then keep a photo of the person near you, glancing at it before you sleep. Or if you're looking for a breakthrough on a design project on which you're working, have some of its elements close at hand.

- Given that dreams are containers of mood and emotion, you may find that listening to music, reading a poem, or looking at artwork before sleep is a wonderful way to help incubate your dream. It's important, of course, to select it intentionally, as you want it to be relaxing yet revelatory, something that lulls you sweetly to drift off to dreamland.

- As fragrance is a powerful catalyst of mood and memory, using specific essential oils in your bedroom may help induce dream content that's in alignment with your focus. For example, if your query is centered on your sex life, use a sultry fragrance like ylang ylang. Or if you're looking for insights related to your childhood, and rosemary reminds you of that time, use that in your aromatherapy diffuser. (For more on using essential oils, see page 46.)

- Remind yourself that you will remember your dream when you awaken, and practice a visualization exercise that will encourage the incubation. For example, you can do a quick meditation in which you bring the following image to your mind's eye: you, waking up in the morning, with clear dream recall, writing down what you remember in your bedside journal, being content that you are filled with the clarity that you had sought.

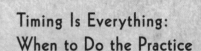

Timing Is Everything: When to Do the Practice

Dream incubation works best when you can carve out the time for it, and when you feel a sense of steadfast determination that you are truly interested in the answers that this practice may yield. Therefore, it's not necessarily something you need to do every night. You want to do it when you have time and focus. So, if your schedule is such that you need to rush out of bed the next morning, save it for another day. Also, given that you want to have this be as attentive and intentional as possible, it's better to not do this practice on nights that you've been up late, have had a few more drinks than usual, or are otherwise distracted.

Other Incubation Applications

The pre-sleep intentionality that's inherent in this dream-incubation practice is also one that is used for other aims. For example, if you suffer from nightmares, before going to sleep you could tell your mind that your dreams will be pleasant and full of ease. Those who lucid dream use a form of incubation wherein they remind and encourage themselves that they will be able to recognize that they are in a dream once they enter that state. Dream incubation can also be a practice that you modify for your children when working with them and their dreams. For more on nightmares, see chapter 8; on lucid dreaming, chapter 9; and on children's dreams, chapter 19.

POSSIBLE CHALLENGES

Of course, it's possible that you may not remember your dream. Keep at it, perhaps seeing if any of the dream-recall techniques in chapter 12 can help you better remember your oneiric visions. Relatedly, what if your dream, no matter from which angle you perceived it, had nothing to do with your question? That can definitely happen, so don't be dismayed. In research studies, many participants didn't have success inducing focused dream content on the first try, and for some, it took weeks of practice. If that's the case, continue to focus upon your question for several days to see if something comes through. If it doesn't, then trust that and your inner knowledge; perhaps it's just not the right moment for the answer to be revealed.

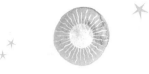

CHAPTER TWELVE

RECALLING YOUR DREAMS

As we know, dreams are mysterious and magical, inspiring and informative. They can provide us with answers to questions alluding us, give us awareness that may bolster our well-being, awe us with their imaginal wonder, and offer us access to a deep well of wisdom — that is, if we can remember them. Whether we want to undertake a concentrated dreamwork practice or we're just curious as to what was included in our nighttime musings, we need to remember our oneiric visions, bringing them to the awareness of our conscious mind. As much as there may be disagreement as to what dreams signify, there is definitely one thing that most everyone agrees upon: it's challenging to remember your dreams and not have them slip away.

One of the most frustrating things is waking up in the morning, being able to sense that you had a dream, and yet be unable to recall it. The dream feels at once so close, yet so far away. You know it's there, just right around some proverbial corner in your mind, and yet, you can't access it. Similarly frustrating — or for some, perhaps more so — is waking up with memory of a dream fragment, only to have it vaporize from your mind just moments later. To think that epics of reverie have occurred, to which you were present in a very special way, but which you can't bring to conscious memory, can be baffling, let alone disheartening. It feels like a tease, a cruel trick that someone is playing on us. Still, thankfully, there are tips and tricks that can help us more readily recall our dreams. Before we explore these, let's try to understand why it often seems like such a formidable task to remember our dreams.

Why Are Dreams So Hard to Remember?

Greek mythology offers us one vantage point, an archetypal lens through which to perceive this oneiric enigma. It turns out that the Greek god of sleep, Hypnos, lived in a cave by the River Lethe, a waterway famous for being a stream that inspired oblivion, as anyone who drank from it would soon forget their past. Reflecting this, it's as if when we sleep, we enter into a cavern in which forgetting seems to be the status quo and a natural part of the terrain we traverse. Mythology aside, let's look at some modern-day reflections that may help us understand why remembering our dreams can be so challenging.

IT'S A MATTER OF TIME

Part of the reason that we forget our dreams may come down to a numbers game. It's been noted that our dreams disappear rather quickly when we transition from sleeping to waking. On average, within 5 minutes, we forget 50 percent of what we dream; within 10 minutes, only 10 percent may remain. Given this, if we don't set about to capture them soon after we awaken, they may drift away and be exceptionally difficult to reclaim.

DREAMS DEFY THE ORDINARY

We spend much of our waking days using left-brain thinking, addressing and processing ideas in a rational, analytical, and linear fashion. But dreams are different, bastions of the fantastical that often defy daytime-consensus reality. As such, it may take effort for us to get our head around what we just perceived, not necessarily readily having the words to describe the seemingly illogical events that we just witnessed. Plus, while some dreams may feature conversations, our oneiric adventures are heavily visual. For many people, trying to quickly translate these visual images — which may seem nonsensical, and therefore, hard to define into words — may be a difficult experience. We struggle to do so, and as time ticks away, our ability to remember them slips away.

THE BARRIER OF OUR BRAIN CHEMISTRY

The work of sleep scientists may help us to further understand just why it's so difficult to remember our dreams. There are certain neurotransmitters (brain chemicals) necessary to transform short-term memories into long-term ones; some of these — including norepinephrine — are at a very low level while we're dreaming, therefore creating an innate blockade to having our nighttime visions etched into our mind. The shift of brain chemistry, and the concurrent fluctuations in the activity of different brain regions that occurs as we move between waking, sleeping, and dreaming, may provide us with clues about why our physiology inherently restricts us from readily remembering our dreams.

THE COST OF COMPROMISED SLEEP

The dreams that arrive in the early morning hours are thought to be more vivid and complex, given that at this point, the REM sleep stage — known for producing more highly activated and visual dreams — lasts longer. Therefore, those who are short sleepers, including those who have sleep-maintenance insomnia and wake up early and can't fall back to sleep, may miss out on these dreams. And since their heightened vividness and emotional saliency make them so stirring and memorable, it may be that we're not remembering our dreams because we're not having these highly impressionable ones.

THE STRENGTH OF AVOIDANCE

Some posit that dreams are repositories for the thoughts and feelings that we brush aside during the day, those that we avoid facing. If our dreams contain unacknowledged aspects of ourselves that we tried to initially avoid, it would make sense that we may have built-in defenses that would work hard to keep them at bay from our conscious mind. It then follows that if we want to keep the premise of "out of sight, out of mind" alive, we could create resistance to remembering our dreams. Relatedly, if we had nightmares as a child, or other experiences that had us associating dreams with negative experiences, we may do whatever we can to try to push away our oneiric memories so that we don't have to encounter them.

Who's More Apt to Remember Their Dreams?

Some people can regularly recall the finest details of their dreams, while others awaken with no memory at all, even questioning whether they've had a dream. What determines whether someone can remember their dreams is something that medical researchers have been interested in for quite some time, with their work unearthing numerous significant and interesting discoveries. Understanding what may differentiate those who are high- versus low-recallers can be of great guidance if we want to further forge our oneiric recollection skills and take our recall game to the next level. Characteristics of those who more regularly recall their dreams include the following.

THEY ACKNOWLEDGE THE VALUE OF THEIR DREAMS

Not surprisingly, those who revere their dreams and accept them as an integral part of their life remember them more often. Those in cultures around the world, and throughout history, that value dreams as an important periscope into knowledge display a greater ability to bring them forth into the waking world. And those who regularly share their dreams with others — whether it be their partner, friends, relatives, or community members — have been found to have greater access to their dreams. Similarly, research suggests that those who have more confidence that they can remember them actually do.

THEY ARE MORE SENSITIVE AND OPEN TO NEW EXPERIENCES

High dream recallers may also be more likely to have certain personality traits. The characteristic known as openness — in which someone is more motivated and capable of adapting to new experiences — has been linked to better dream recall. Those who are sensitive and have thinner personal boundaries have also been found to remember their dreams more often. Not surprisingly, those who struggle to find words to describe their feelings seem to recall their dreams less frequently.

THEY ARE IMAGINATIVE

Those who are creative and imaginative also tend to remember their dreams more often. Since they contain a concentrated pictorial element, it's not surprising that visual learners, creatives, and those more sensitive to aesthetics have been found to have better recall.

THEY ARE INTROSPECTIVE

Dreamers who regularly tune in to their inner world have been found to have better recall. These include people who have meditation and contemplative practices, as well as those who are in therapy. People who are highly oriented to their imaginal life — whether through daydreaming or letting their imaginations soar — are also more apt to remember their dreams.

THEY GET ADEQUATE SLEEP

It would also make sense that those who get more sleep are more apt to remember their dreams for the sheer reason that there are more of them to possibly recall. Plus, as we've seen, early morning REM periods are longer and provide us with an extended opportunity to have vivid dreams. Given that such dreams may be more intricate, they may also be more memorable.

THEY TEND TO BE YOUNGER AND FEMALE

Research has found that dream recall peaks in early adulthood and declines from there on, notably lower in older age. Whether this is biologically based or a reflection of a decreasing interest in dreams and their introspective nature is not clear. Women seem to remember their dreams more than men do; the reason for this is uncertain, although it could relate to the fact that women, generally speaking, tend to be more emotionally focused than men and seek to understand their feelings (something that dreams can offer).

General Recall Strategies

Based upon these research findings, we can create strategies that may help our dream recall.

BELIEVE IN THE VALUE OF YOUR DREAMS

The fact that you're reading this book already puts you at an advantage, since it reflects your interest — or at least a concentrated curiosity — to more deeply connect with your dreams and all that they may offer you. Continuing to advocate for their role in your life and well-being may help you to remember them more often. Additionally, being grateful for what they reveal — whether something practical or just fascinating — is a sign of reverence, which we have seen is a factor that helps to amplify recall. Similarly, following breakthrough solutions that a dream contains lets it know that you honor it.

HAVE CONFIDENCE YOU'LL REMEMBER THE DREAM

When you go to sleep at night, tell yourself you will remember your oneiric visions. Think of yourself as someone who not only has dreams — we all do — but someone who can bring memories of them forward into the waking world. Even on days that you don't remember anything or even very little, remind yourself that that's OK and doesn't mean that you won't access more tomorrow. On those days, still continue to make an entry into your dream journal, noting, "I had dreams, although I don't remember them right now."

GET GOOD SLEEP

You can add remembering your dreams to the list of the many benefits that having adequate sleep yields (see page 26 for a survey of others). Those who have sufficient sleep invariably have more REM sleep, and a greater concentration of the more vivid and memorable dreams that occur in this slumber stage. Make a concerted effort to aim for your target sleep goals; for most adults, that's 7-plus hours each night.

CURATE YOUR CREATIVITY

Exposing yourself to more visual images during the day will help exercise the associated part of your brain, enhancing your facility to experience the world this way. Appreciate the image itself, perceiving all of its nuances. Allocate time to writing about some images you see, describing them as clearly as you can; this will allow you to further develop a link between what you see and the words that can describe it, a skill inherently important for capturing your dreams. Also, inspire your right brain by reading poetry. This type of prose is usually nonlinear in its wayfinding. As such, it's similar to dreams and may allow your mind to start thinking more in this manner.

CONNECT TO YOUR FEELINGS

Being more connected to our feelings has many benefits, not the least being that it may help us to remember our dreams. If we're open to the emotions that may arise, knowing we have the capacity to deal with what may come, it helps us better remember what was carried forth in our oneiric visions.

Similarly, spending more time being introspective may also be of benefit. Take a quiet walk, relax in a bath while listening to music, let yourself daydream. If you don't have a meditation practice, start one.

BE MORE OPEN-MINDED

Being more adaptable, curious, and open to adventure is a way of orienting that has many benefits, including greater oneiric recall. Try to be more amenable to surprises and detours (something with which dreams are filled), knowing that they sometimes put you on a path that yields unexpected, and beneficial, experiences and insights.

TALK ABOUT YOUR DREAMS

Find friends, family, or colleagues to talk to about your dreams. See if your partner or your child is interested in a morning check-in, with each person asking the other how their dreams were. Explore dream groups in your area, or start one (see chapter 15 for more information on this subject). Having an encouraging social context will help you to remember them more often.

Tips for Enhanced Dream Recall

Try the tips below if you are having trouble remembering
your dreams.

- Don't judge any images that come forth. Just allow them to arise.
  Resist resisting what may surface. In general, at this point, you don't want to play
  editor; rather, you want to assume the role of an inviting audience, witnessing all
  that is occurring.

- Remember that you may recall a story line or perhaps one or several images, or both.
  One is not better than the other: be open to what comes through. If you remember
  even one detail, don't discount its value. Stay with it. Let it marinate.

- Tune in to how you feel when you awaken. Even if you can't access images, knowing the
  feeling state that the dream inspired is of great value. Tune in to how the dream felt.

- If you're not readily able to access dream images or a story line, scan through the faces
  of people to whom you're emotionally connected. They may have been represented
  in your dream, and this may trigger a memory. Additionally, since many dreams are
  strongly influenced by our recent waking experiences, survey your previous day and
  see if any event that occurred sparks a dream memory.

- Once images and/or a story line appear, go back over them again and again in your
  mind, to assist in etching them into your memory. Remember that while the first set
  of impressions you receive are, in and of themselves, exceptionally valuable, they will
  likely lead to your ability to mine for others that are connected to them.

- No matter how much you remember, document it. If you don't remember anything, just
  note that. By doing so, you'll emphasize your belief that, in fact, you do have dreams.
  This will allow for the unbroken continuation of your dream-capturing routine.

- Create a set of small note cards that contain the name of the images, symbols, places,
  or words that occur frequently in your dreams. After you've spent your first several
  minutes awake being quiet with your eyes closed, you can then look at the cards and
  see if they trigger a memory of anything that occurred in your dream.

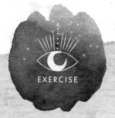

Recall Rituals

Here are some time-honored practices that can heighten your ability to consciously connect to the dreams you've had.

Before Bed

1 Make sure that the tools you're going to use capture your dreams — whether paper and pen, audio recorder, or something else — are easily accessible by your bedside.

2 Some people find that reflecting upon their day backward helps them to then go back into their dreams when they wake up. To do so, as you're relaxing before you doze off, visualize yourself in bed, then think about what you did just before getting into bed, what occurred before then, and before then, taking yourself on a quick tour of your day, from finish to start. This practice can help you in the morning, as you'll be readily primed to take a back-in-time orientation and look to see what oneiric visions just recently arose in your mind.

3 As you relax to fall asleep, tell yourself that you will have dreams while you're sleeping, and that you will remember them in the morning.

4 Practice dream incubation (see chapter 11), in which you contemplate the insights and solutions that you'd like your dream to include. In addition to helping you to access key problem-solving and creative insights, this technique hones intention, which can enhance recall. Remind yourself that when you wake up in the morning, you will relax in bed for a few minutes so that you can capture your dream.

Upon Awakening

1 Be leisurely when you awaken. Don't jump out of bed, nor feel a sense of pressure that you need to begin your day immediately. You're still in the liminal space between sleeping and waking, and the connection to the dream is still strong.

2 This can help you to access and bring them back to consciousness. Remember, the first 5 to 10 minutes provide you with the most opportune time for recalling your dreams.

3 If the position you generally sleep in is different than the one in which you wake up, gently go back to your slumbering position, as this will connect you to what's known as state-dependent memory. Doing so may help you to access your dreams.

CHAPTER THIRTEEN

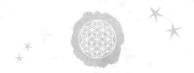

DOCUMENTING YOUR DREAMS

Now that you're armed with strategies to enhance your dream recall, let's explore the next important stage in working with your dreams: capturing and documenting them. For some people, remembering their dreams each night is rewarding enough. Just the process of recalling them and giving them voice satisfies a desire to acknowledge what the dream brought forth. Others like to collect and organize their dreams in a capsule, a dream journal in which they can take up residence, and from which they can be read and reread, worked through to yield the wealth of insights that they can offer.

For those who like to collect them in a cache, some like to write down their dreams directly into their journals as they're remembering them. Others, though, find that they like to have an intermediate step, one in which they first capture their dream and then transcribe it into their journal afterward, finding this helps them be more methodical as they unpack their dream's meaning. Regardless of whether you're a one- or multi-step dream journaler, this chapter will provide you with tips and tidbits that will augment this process for you. Remember that when it comes to dreamwork, there's no one-size-fits-all approach. Explore the techniques within this chapter, seeing which ones may serve you in your dreamwork practice.

Capturing Your Dreams

Using the dream-catching strategies discussed in the previous chapter, you'll be able to tap into initial memories of your nighttime visions. As they coalesce in your mind, the next step is to glean and capture them, shuttling what you've recollected — whether an entire story line or just even an image or a feeling — out of your mind and into documented form. Writing down dreams is the standard approach, but numerous other strategies also can be helpful, depending upon the unique style through which you process information.

Regardless of which method you choose, it's important to not judge or edit yourself when you're trying to bring forth your dreams. Record everything that comes to you, whether or not it seems to make sense. Don't worry about getting the sequence right when you first record your dreams; just document everything that you recall initially, knowing that you will string things together in a more formal way later on. Even if what you're remembering doesn't seem especially cogent, you may find that these threads of memory eventually will lead you down a path that connects you to other details that you didn't initially access. This is one of the reasons that many people find it beneficial to record their dreams in two stages: (1) the initial capturing stage, when you first wake up; and (2) the subsequent phase when you document them, transferring your recollections to a journal and further organizing and working with them. Not feeling the pressure to get your dream first scribed in a certain systematic (or even tidy) way will give you more freedom and disengage the censoring you may be otherwise inclined to do. This allows you unencumbered connection to your dream memory while it's still fresh in your mind.

Also, try not to interpret your dreams as you're first trying to capture them, as this, too, can thwart your ability to remember precious insights. There will be lots of time to analyze and interpret them later. This first phase is the fact-finding stage and we want to mine and recover as much treasure as we can. Here are several approaches for initially capturing your dreams. Unless you have a tried-and-true method, consider experimenting with these, seeing which works better for you. Also, you don't have to choose just one. You may find that a combination works for you, or that some fit better with certain styles of dreams or at different times in your life.

WRITING

Most people capture their dreams by jotting them down on paper. And while writing them immediately into a dream journal may be standard fare, as previously noted, some people find this approach to have a restrictive drawback; this may arise from numerous factors, including that their middle-of-the-night handwriting may not necessarily be all that legible and in a form that they want to have preserved forever in their journal.

Additionally, feeling that they want their journal to be neat and orderly may have them place undue pressure on themselves when writing down their dream images, which could stifle the spontaneity of what is arising.

A great workaround? Instead of first writing in your journal, record your dreams on paper that you keep by your bedside. This can be a small pad, notebook, index cards, a loose sheet of paper — anything that has a shape and size that allows you to easily write. Record all that you can on this paper, and then later transcribe it into your dream journal.

Of course, you'll need a good writing instrument. Have one that writes really easily, in which you take pleasure using. Make sure before you go to bed that it has ink in it, or if it's a pencil, that it's sharpened. After all, you want to avoid the commonplace frustration of having access to a bevy of dream memories ready to be transcribed, only to not be able to do so because of a dried-up pen or blunted pencil.

Given that you may awaken in the middle of the night and want to write your dreams, having a light source is also important. Best is a hands-free headlight, a pen that has a light attached, or a book light attached to your notebook. The light should be strong enough to see by, yet not too illuminative to be jarring or stimulating, to yourself or your bed partner.

Some people find that typing their dreams into the notes section of their phone or tablet works as a good method. Others, however, find that there's more of a chance for spelling mistakes to occur, and that it ends up making the dream record less decipherable. Plus, if you end up spending time correcting typos or erroneous autocorrects along the way, you may find that it eats into the precious moments you initially have while your dreams are still fresh in your mind. In addition, if you're logging dreams in the middle of the night, you want to avoid the melatonin-stymieing blue light from tech screens, as it can lead to subsequent sleep disruption. The other disadvantage to this approach is reflected in the benefit of handwriting: the process of putting pen to paper helps us to allocate things to memory better than does typing. All said, though, if you've found this system works for you, then continue to use it.

DRAWING

Sometimes it's really hard to capture dreams in writing; after all, they are so visual. In these cases, give yourself the freedom to draw, as it's a great way to fish out dream images and feelings. You can draw anything from the dream — you need not limit yourself to just diagramming an image. You may even find that scribbling lines on a paper helps you to capture a scene's layout. Or, if you remember a certain color that casts a hue throughout the dream, you can use a colored pencil or marker to represent it.

Doodling is really helpful, too, as sometimes you may not be able to access images, but can readily tap into the feelings elicited by the dream and express them in uniquely formed lines and shapes. Since dreams are often not linear and don't mirror the arrangement of space to which we're accustomed, doodling them may give you more boundless freedom to connect to them.

A pictorial approach can also be used to express the sequence of events, drawing small scenes one after the other. You may find that sometimes just allowing yourself to draw a shape that feels related to your dream will trigger a greater memory of what occurred, whether at the moment or later on. Remember that what you draw need not be a work of art, or even something recognizable. Don't judge yourself; just let yourself be free. Don't worry about being a Picasso; whatever you can get on paper has exceptional value.

AUDIO RECORDING

Even if you're a fast writer, sometimes you may find that the pace of your writing is slower than necessary to document all of the details that come forth when you remember a dream. A great workaround for this is to audio record your oneiric memories. You don't even need to get a new device, as many phones come with a preinstalled voice-recording app. And if yours doesn't, don't worry: there are scores that can be purchased and downloaded, some even for free. It's amazing how much more quickly most people can speak their dreams than write them. And since we know that time is key, because they dissipate so quickly, recording them may help you to access and preserve more of them.

There may be another benefit as well; after all, when we first awaken from slumber, and our muscles are regaining the coordination they lost during sleep, our handwriting may not be at its peak. Our voice, though, even if it's muffled, is still pretty recognizable. Perhaps you've had that experience of feeling really excited that you remembered a dream and wrote it down, only to later feel so frustrated when you were unable to make heads or tails of it; audio recording it is a way to sidestep this possibility.

For privacy purposes, you likely won't want to have your recorded dreams on your phone for too long, unless you regularly use a password to guard access. As such, you can even opt to send it right away to your computer, or upload it to cloud storage, and then erase it before you transcribe it in your journal. Don't forget to give it a title that includes the date so that you can readily find it.

This approach may be tricky if you share a bed with someone and you awaken before they do. Not only, of course, will speaking out loud rouse them, but it may also infringe upon your privacy. As such, you may need to quickly steal away to the bathroom or another secluded spot to record your dreams. This approach may work fine in the morning, although it might not end up being the best strategy for middle-of-the-night recalls, given that shuffling out of bed could be jarring and impinge upon your ability to get back to sleep. If that's the case for you, then you may want to opt instead for jotting or drawing your middle-of-the-night dream memories.

VIDEO RECORDING

Some people like to capture some of their dreams in video format. With this method, you get to not only record the audio but also some of the visual components of your oneiric visions. Video also allows you to reflect the emotions that the dream evoked through capturing your facial expressions or movements. Remember, you don't have to keep the video for time immemorial; it's just a tool for you to document the initial memories of your dreams. Once you transcribe the video into words, you can then delete it. No special equipment is needed for this method; just use the video feature on your smartphone's camera.

DREAM JOURNALING APPS

Another way to document your dreams is to do so with an app, which you can use on either your phone or tablet. The features of apps range, but at their heart, they include a diary in which you can type your dream. Many also include the ability to add tags to further code them. There are also apps designed for lucid dreamers, which not only feature tips and techniques but also alarms and notification functions that can remind you to do reality checks (see chapter 9 for more on lucid dreaming). If you want to tap into a community of virtual dreamers, some apps feature a database of users' dreams that you can search through to read and/or comment upon.

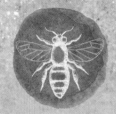

Say Your Dreams Aloud

Sometimes, saying a dream aloud helps you to better remember it. If you share a bed with someone, and it feels right, you can share your dream with each other when you wake up. Speaking your dream can help to make it conscious and commit it to memory. Plus, sharing dreams may be a sweet ritual to do with someone with whom you are intimate. This ritual is a nod to ones done in more traditional communities, wherein dreams would be listened to by the tribe or a trusted advisor.

Capture What You Can

There may be times when you remember an epic amount of your dream and have the time to write it down immediately. There may be other times, though, when you don't have that luxury, either because you can't access that much of your dream or you need to get out of bed pretty quickly. There may also be times when you need to further jog your memory a bit to be able to net even a whisper of what transpired. If you don't have much time and/or you can't initially remember that much, still, try to spend a couple of minutes to write down what you remember. Consider doing one of these exercises, which will help you to scribe some oneiric souvenirs.

Seven Words

Write down seven words that feel connected to your dream. These could be related to things that happened, symbols that appeared, or the tone that wove itself through. Aim for seven words, but if you can't access that target, write as many as you can.

Connect to the Feeling

Jot down how you feel upon waking, what your mood is like. And if you can remember the feeling tone of your dream, note that as well.

Body Orientation

Scan your body and see whether your attention focuses in on any specific area. Consider whether your dream featured that part, or parts, of your body as a key image. Document any pertinent information.

The 4 Ws

Quickly jot the signature aspects of your dream, from a Who, Where, What, and When perspective.

Who: The main characters

Where: Description of the location or locations

What: A few notes about what transpired

When: Identify the time — whether in general as past, present, future — or more specifically, if you can, in which the dream took place.

Dream Documenting

Putting all your dreams in one place — a journal, for example — allows you to keep them organized so that you can return to them at a later time, reviewing and finding more meaning within them, whether in a single dream or across several of them. And even if you don't return to your dreams regularly, or ever again, just knowing that they are recorded imbues them with reverence and a sense of validity. It encourages them to take on the feel of a documentary of your life, or part of your life.

And there is also the other benefit of this two-stage process, where you initially capture your dreams and then later transcribe them in a journal: it gives you another opportunity to remember possibly forgotten details. The process of transferring them from their initial state — whether written, drawn, voice recorded, or video recorded — gives you an additional chance to bring forth more possibly forgotten facets of the dream, allowing you to unearth more awareness as to what it revealed than you may have initially considered.

As you'll see in the next chapter, it's recommended to have a section within each journal entry where you write your unedited notes and recollections. You will use these initial memories that you captured in the steps just outlined to further detail and decipher your dreams. Here are some tips for documenting your dreams, transferring them from their originally captured form to your journal repository.

WHEN

Have this practice be one that has as much consistency as feels right. Consider blocking off some time each day to doing so. If that doesn't work for you, you can allocate several days a week to transcribe your dream notes into your journal. If you do it each day, it can be just after you've captured them, or later on. You can do this step separate from the next one, in which you further work and decode the dream (discussed in chapter 14), or during the same time frame.

Allocate a period of time in which you have adequate ability to do this. Make sure you won't have interruptions. Prepare some coffee or tea, play some music, and/or light candles. Do whatever feels right to make this a relaxing and enjoyable practice. This process can take as much or as little time as you want and have. Don't feel pressured to consistently have it be a dedicated activity. Even just spending 5 minutes to initially document your dreams in your journal will be a significant step in the process.

WHERE

While you can do this activity anywhere, consider allocating a dedicated space to doing it, as this will make it more of a ritual. It can be at your desk, the kitchen table, a chair in the living room, a cushion by your dream altar, your bathtub, or any other place that feels nurturing to you. If you associate this spot with reflection work, once you arrive there, you will feel more attuned to slowing down, being inwardly quiet, and getting into a dreamier space. Have it be someplace where you can have privacy and quiet, whether it's a room that has a door or a spot that you know won't be used by anyone else in the family at a certain time. Keep your dreamwork supplies there; this, of course, includes your journal, but may also include items such as writing and drawing instruments (markers, colored pencils, pastels, and the like), as well as scrapbooking/collaging items (such as magazines, scissors, glue, etc.) if you want to have your journal feature multi-media representations of your dreams.

HOW

The first step is to transcribe or add your dream recollections to your journal in an unfiltered way. As previously noted, it's always good to have a section in your journal that just features the raw material, the original capture, of your dream. (See dream journal design ideas in chapter 14.)

If you captured your dream in written words, transcribe them in your journal. If you captured your dream in pictures, you can do one of two things: redraw them in your journal or affix the originals with tape.

If you captured your dream in audio form, transcribe what you said into words. If you're using a computer-based dream journal, you can even use transcription software to do so, although make sure to read it over afterward. This is important for two reasons: you don't want there to be any misinterpretations, and you want the opportunity to reconnect with your dreams at this point.

To Sleep, or to Record a Dream?

Given that most of us have four to five periods of vivid dream potential through a night's sleep, there are numerous opportunities to capture our dreams. Some dreamers may have no qualms about grabbing their journal in the middle of the night should they arise mid-sleep to write down the whispers of their oneiric visions. And lucid dreamers who practice the Wake Back to Bed method (see page 102) may even intentionally set their alarm clocks to wake them up in the early morning hours; this way, they can not only record a dream, but also stay awake and practice techniques that may foster their lucidity. And yet, there may be times that you arise from a dream and would rather turn over to go back to sleep than turn on the light and write in your journal. There's no right or wrong; do what feels aligned with your dream inquiry quest, as well as the ways in which you know you need to tap into your rest.

If you captured your dream in video, transcribe the audio portion into words. If you're using a paper dream journal, describe in words the movements you made or the facial expressions you used. If you're using a digital dream journal, you may be able to import the video and integrate it as part of the entry record.

As you begin to transfer your notes, you may find that you can remember more of the dream. One image may lead to another, or you may see how some of the things you recall string together with others.

Next Steps

After you've transcribed your initial recollections in your dream journal, you can begin to survey your dreams to further access the layers of wisdom that they have afforded you. One of the key steps in decoding your dreams — understanding individual ones as well as groups of them — is to identify the different components that they include, as well as attributes that they have. This is something that you can easily do by organizing the pages of your dream journal in a certain way, and something that we'll explore in the next chapter.

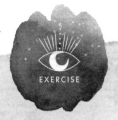

EXERCISE

More Documenting Tips

As you're documenting your dreams, you have yet another opportunity to remember more of them. Here are some additional dream-mining activities to consider:

- If you remember a movement that occurred in your dream, act it out. This proprioceptive experience may help trigger other dream memories.

- If a line from a song appeared in your dream, listen to the entire song to see whether it jogs your memory of your dream or gives you more context as to why it was included.

- If you use the tarot as a tool for divining insights, pick a card while intentioning that it will help you connect to something in your dream you may not have yet remembered. Survey the card and look at its entire gestalt, as well as the individual images, design dynamics, the name of the card, and even its number. It's easiest to do this exercise using only the twenty-two Major Arcana cards.

CHAPTER FOURTEEN

USING A DREAM JOURNAL

For many, their dream journal is the centerpiece of their dreamwork practice, a capsule in which their oneiric odysseys are preserved. A dream journal serves as a looking-glass chronicle through which we can reconnect to the hopes, wishes, fears, and concerns that channel through our minds and hearts, which are uniquely revealed during the night when we sleep and dream. Our dream journals are replete with autobiographical reflections that help us to know ourselves better, all the while also having us remember the exquisite power that emerges when we tap into our imaginal mind. In addition to being a coffer of self-awareness treasures, our dream journals not only serve as the destination for our insights, but also as a tool that helps us to discover the wisdom that our dreams yield.

The Array of Dream Journals

There are numerous dream journals available. While some feature beautiful covers and inspirational quotes, there are others that are designed to help encourage you to remember your dreams and record them in ways in which you can access their deeper levels. Some come complete with section headings ready-made for you to scribe the date, title, and some visual notes, while others include journaling prompts, checkboxes to help you describe the dream, and spaces dedicated to both recording and reflecting upon it. If you've not found a dream journal that's visually appealing, helps you to stay motivated, and also acts as a guide to help unearth what your dreams may mean, there's another option: you can create your own. It's not difficult nor time-consuming, and it can be one of the most powerful steps you can take to connect to the heart of the wisdom that your dreams contain.

All it requires is creating different sections in your journal pages, areas that help you to organize some of your dream details in a way that mirrors your interests and meets your needs. It's a powerful tool to help you zero in on the numerous facets of your dreams and further understand just what they may mean. This chapter will give you some tips and strategies that can boost your journaling practice to take your dreamwork to the next level.

Types of Journals

Before we get into the details on how to make a customized journal that addresses the things that you're most interested in assessing and analyzing, let's start at the beginning, and consider what type of book to use. There are generally two basic options from which to choose. Regardless of which you select, choose a size that will work best for you in terms of providing you a good amount of space to write. Even if you don't use it all, not feeling constrained may open up the channel to your memory; it's a way of sending a message to your subconscious mind that you know that there is something vast that wants to be shared and understood, and that you're giving yourself adequate space where it can be documented. By doing so, you're imparting a greater sense of possibility and encouragement, which can inspire a better ability to understand the vast layers of your dream.

NOTEBOOK

There are a range of notebook possibilities from which to choose. You could use a simple spiral-bound book. Or, you could opt for a bound notebook; if so, find one that lies flat when opening it, as you'll soon see how instrumental working with facing pages is. For most people, blank pages offer more freedom of expression than ones that are lined, allowing them to also have a space to draw or doodle if they choose. Others prefer those that are dotted, as this helps them to make lines to readily demarcate different sections. See what works best for your particular journaling style. Given that you'll want to number the pages, if it already has page numbers printed on it, that can be a plus. As you'll soon see, if you choose to use a notebook, you'll be making space on each page for different sections in which you will fill in an array of information related to your dreams.

BINDER BOOK

Another approach is to create templated pages on the computer, print them out, three-hole punch them, and keep them in a binder. You'd print them on two sides, with each page having a different layout on the front and back (you'll see examples of this in the coming pages). This allows you to not only record and organize different aspects of your dreams but also take advantage of there being facing pages with which to work. Like with the notebook option, make sure that the binder opens flat for ease of use.

Dream Journal Page Designs

Designing your own dream journal is not only easy and creative, but it can also help you to access deeper levels of insights. Whether you want a design that lets you capture the basics or a bespoke one that allows you to track a variety of different dream variables that may be of interest, in the following pages you'll find suggestions on how to organize your journal to optimize your dreamwork.

As you'll see, in each of these layout options, I suggest that instead of having each night's dream featured on subsequent pages, that you allocate two facing pages — one of the left and one on the right side of your journal — for each dream. Not only does this expansive space give your psyche a sense of freedom so that it doesn't feel limited as to what it can capture and document, but it also inspires your ability to make more connections. One of my favorite ways to use these facing pages, and which serves as the foundation for my approach, is to document initial memories of a dream on the left-side page and scribe reflections on the dream's significance on the right-side page. Being able to see both your dream memories and your reflections at once enables a dialogue that not only engages your mind, but can also bring through originally forgotten dream details. It's a much easier and more efficient approach than having to flip back and forth between pages that contain information on the same dream. And there's another benefit: if you're someone who likes to write their dream directly into their journal rather than take an intermediate step (as we discussed in the last chapter), having a dedicated space that's separate from any evaluation or reflection can help you keep your dream journal more organized.

BASIC JOURNAL DESIGN

The basic dream journal design suits many people quite well. For the basic one, you just need a space for the following information, which you arrange on facing pages.

Date: Including the date you had the dream is, of course, essential. Given that we often don't know the exact moment we had a dream, and we may be interested in understanding our dream in the context of the previous day's events, consider including the dates of both the evening you went to bed and the morning you awoke in your journal.

Memories: Allocate a good portion of the left-hand page for documenting all that you recalled from your dream. You can either write directly in here as you're recalling your dream or transcribe what you originally wrote elsewhere, or what you audio or video recorded when you first arose.

Reflections: This is the section in which you document what you feel the dream signifies. It's where you record your ongoing thoughts on the different layers of the dream, and what message it may be offering you.

Page Number: Numbering the pages will allow you to create a Table of Contents so that you can readily rediscover a dream you had (for more on this, see page 166).

Title: Giving your dream a title can help you to further distill its meaning and significance. You can also use it in your journal's Table of Contents when cataloging your dreams. Additionally, giving it a title is another opportunity to express your creativity in your dreamwork.

On the next pages, you'll see an example of a basic journal design layout. You can either draw these sections in your notebook journal, or if you're making templates to print out — or use in a digital journal — you can use them as the basis of your design.

Memories

DATE: _____

PAGE:

Reflections

TITLE: _____

BESPOKE JOURNAL DESIGN

While the basic design works great, you may find that you want to capture other details related to your dreams. Including additional categories of information will not only make your dream journal richer, but it will also further enhance your ability to see what your dreams may be revealing. Plus, it's a great system to help you understand patterns that may weave throughout your dreams (for more on this, see page 162).

Here are some ideas of categories that you can include in your dream journal. Experiment with the ones that seem most interesting; you need not use all of them. Try different ones at different times to see which ones help you to best connect with your dreams and understand what they mean. Of course, this isn't an exhaustive list. As you continue to work with your dreams, you may find additional subjects that are of interest that you may want to include.

Feelings

Dreams often have an emotional tone. Sometimes it's even easier to connect with the feeling tone of the dream than it is to recover the who, what, where, and when details that it featured. Additionally, as our dreams are often related to the processing of opportunities and challenges from our waking life — and the related emotions that they bring forth — what we were feeling before we fell asleep often informs our dreams.

And as we know, the demarcation between dreaming and waking isn't that stringent. Often what is catalyzed in our dreams infuses itself into our waking awareness afterward, sometimes with such tenacity that it feels hard to shake off the emotional residue that a dream imparted. As such, questions that address our feelings may yield interesting insights. Consider adding a section to your journal with the following or similar questions. You can even fill out the first one before you fall asleep.

- How did I feel when I went to bed?
- What feelings arose in my dreams?
- How do I feel upon arising?
- How do I feel after exploring my dreams?

Day's Reflections

Our days and nights weave together, forming the whole tapestry of who we are. Our dreams often reflect our digesting and absorbing the ideas, situations, and feelings that occurred the preceding day. As such, noting daily occurrences may help us to further understand our dreams. Consider including these prompts in your dream journal. You could, of course, answer these questions the night before you go to sleep; just change the orientation of the questions if you do.

- What was I grateful for yesterday?
- What did I worry about yesterday?
- What significant events, if any, transpired yesterday?

Dream Incubation Intention

As we saw in chapter 11, dream incubation is a practice in which you intentionally ask your dream to reveal specific insights that are of import to you. If you are incubating a dream, it's helpful to include the intention in your journal before you go to sleep. This, of course, helps you keep a record of it, and then hones your focus in the morning when you begin to discern what your dream revealed about your query. It also provides another benefit: it's not uncommon to have created the most powerful dream intention as you're unwinding in bed, only to not remember it the next morning.

- Dream incubation intention

Symbols, Images, and Themes

Dreams are rich in symbols, images, and themes that weave throughout. Sometimes we may not even remember the narrative of our dreams, although we can readily recall the iconic visuals that were included within. The images may be those whose meaning is obvious, or they may be rife with substrata of unique meanings that take time to access. These symbols, images, and themes may include anything in the dream that you found striking, whether obtusely mundane or bizarrely out of the ordinary. Note any colors or numbers that may have appeared. If you remember seeing or hearing words, record those as well.

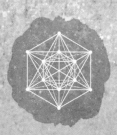

Digital Dream Journals

Traditionally, a reference to a dream journal infers a paper book, whether one that is hard- or spiral-bound. These allow you to write and draw by hand, as well as customize with collages or stickers, and include found objects that feel connected to a dream. However, a dream journal doesn't have to be analog. It can also be created on a digital medium. You can create one using your computer's word-processing software or an online platform that allows you to weave words with digital media.

Unpacking the significance of what a dream symbol means can be a fascinating foundation of our dreamwork, as we come to learn how it speaks to us and reflects the complex weave of who we are. As such, consider adding a section in your journal that highlights the symbols and images that were featured in your dreams. You could have themes woven in there or featured as a separate section.

- Symbols and images
- Themes

Outcomes Inspired

As we reflect upon our dreams, we may find that we get some really powerful takeaways. Some of these may even point us toward actions we feel we are ready to embark upon. Including these in your dream journal will serve as another testament to the healing and wisdom-inspiring benefits that dreams have in your life.

- Takeaways
- Outcomes inspired

Sleeping Environment

The more you do dreamwork, the more you may come to see that certain factors influence the type of dreams you have, and their quality and contents. Some of these may center upon your sleeping environs, as well as factors that influenced your slumber. By tracking these, you may begin to see further interlacing patterns that are not only interesting but also informative. For example, you could include such questions as the following in your dream journal.

- How many hours of sleep did I have?

- How was the quality of my sleep?

- What was I thinking about when I went to sleep?

- Where did I sleep?

- With whom did I sleep?

- Did I have sex before I went to sleep?

- Did I awaken in the night?

- At what approximate time did the dream occur?

Lucid Dreaming

If you lucid dream, you can also track important information in your journal that can help to enhance your practice, let alone allow you to document your awareness-filled adventures. This can include not only details of your oneiric journeys, but also the dream signs you recognized and techniques that you used to foster the dream.

- The sign/s that let me recognize I was in a lucid dream
- The lucid-dreaming techniques I used last night

Ancient Dream Journals

Dream journals are anything but a modern invention. The idea of them actually dates back to at least the fifth century, when Synesius of Cyrene wrote about "night books" in *On Dreams*. He also suggested the benefit of combining day journals with dream journals; in Section 12 of his tome, he notes: "We shall therefore see fit to add to what are called 'day books' what we term 'night books,' so as to have records to remind us of the character of each of the two lives concerned."

AstroDreamwork

For those who are interested in weaving together astrological insights with their dreamwork, you can include additional variables in your journal. These may comprise the phase and/or sign of the Moon, the current astrological passages/transits through which you're moving, or anything else that you find provides you clues as to the meaning of your dreams. (See chapter 16 for more on AstroDreamwork.)

- Moon phase
- Moon sign
- Current astrological passages/ transits

The journal layout on pages 164–165 includes several of these categories with spaces wherein you can document your dream incubation intention; symbols, images, and themes; and the outcomes that were inspired. Again, there are a multitude of different categories that you can choose to use when organizing your dream journal.

PATTERN RECOGNITION

Not only does having categorized sections in your dream journal allow you to dig into them deeper, but it also helps you to recognize patterns that may exist. For example, if you track the images that appear in your dreams and also what you were thinking about before you fell asleep, you may be able to recognize that a certain symbol seems likely to appear when your pre-slumber thoughts were centered on a certain subject. As such, its appearance in your dreams may then have you realize that it's serving as a beacon that's symbolizing something about this particular waking-life consideration. This then allows you to approach your dream decoding with fresh insights.

On page 170, you'll see an example of tracking themes, evening thoughts, and a recurring symbol — a crow, in this instance — that may appear in numerous dreams. Through this, we can see patterns that may emerge. In this case, the presence of the crow more often than not relates to dream themes that have to do with movement and shifting elevations, as well as pre-sleep ruminations related to work. By knowing this, next time a crow appears, or we find ourselves moving from one level to another, we may look to our dream to see what it may be revealing about a work situation.

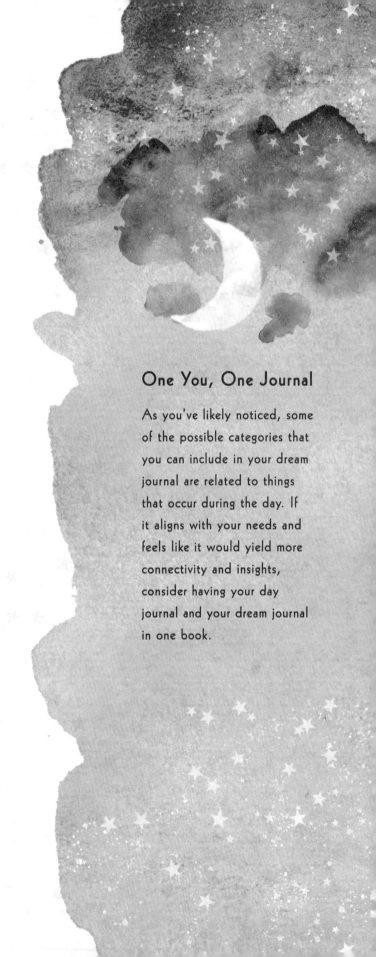

One You, One Journal

As you've likely noticed, some of the possible categories that you can include in your dream journal are related to things that occur during the day. If it aligns with your needs and feels like it would yield more connectivity and insights, consider having your day journal and your dream journal in one book.

Memories

DATE: _____

INTENTION: _____

_____

_____

_____

_____

_____

_____

_____

_____

_____

_____

SYMBOLS/IMAGES: _____

_____

_____

_____

_____

Reflections

TITLE: _____

_____

_____

_____

_____

_____

_____

_____

_____

THEMES: _____

_____

_____

OUTCOMES INSPIRED: _____

_____

_____

PAGE:

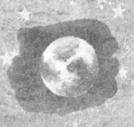

Dreaming Rituals on the Road

As you're always dreaming, you can bring your intentional dreamwork practice with you wherever you go. Your portable dream kit may include your dream journal, dream pillow, and flower essences that aid your slumber. Bring them — especially your journal — along with you in your carry-on, as you never know what elevated visions you may have when at high elevations. Don't forget to pack the things that help you sleep well and have you feel at home wherever you are. If you're unsure about the light and noise environment of your hotel room, bring a sleep mask, earplugs, and/or a mini-pink noise machine with you. You can also still enjoy your favorite centering essential oils on the road: use a travel-size aromatherapy diffuser or pack a premade mist that you can spritz yourself with before sleeping. Also, a dream altar will travel: bring along crystals, candles, sacred images, etc., and create a mini-altar on your hotel nightstand.

You could do this cross-referencing with any variables. For example, if you track themes and Moon phases, you may find that your dreams around the Full Moon are oftentimes more rife with conflict than those at other times of the month. Or, if you observe your feelings and your sleeping environment, you may potentially find a connection between the quality of slumber you had and the emotional tone infused in your dream. How to do this is easy: just create a log in your dream journal where you cross-reference different categories of dream information.

TABLE OF CONTENTS

Allocate several pages in the beginning of your dream journal to create a Table of Contents. It should include basic information, such as the date and title of each dream, as well as the page number. This will allow you to have an ongoing inventory of your dreams. Even just briefly scanning it will provide you with important insights based upon their titles (see pages 168–169).

Other Pages to Include in Your Dream Journal

Here are two other categories that you can include in your dream journal.

Dream Themes

Create a page in your journal where you catalog a list of themes, images, people, and places that commonly appear in your dreams. This way, if you're struggling to remember a dream one morning, you can glance at the theme page to see if it will shake your memory, helping you recall some of the who, what, and where that wove through your dream.

Dream Signs

If you do lucid dreaming, identifying dream signs can be essential in helping you become conscious that you're in a dream. To enhance your facility with recognizing them, it's good to have a list of the places, events, people, or perspectives that commonly appear in your dreams but never occur in your waking life. Go through your journal to find these, and then dedicate a page to a creating a dream-sign list that you can have for handy reference. Review it before you go to sleep, so that you can prime your mind to recognize these when you're in a dream, as this can help to activate your lucidity ability. For more on dream signs, see page 105.

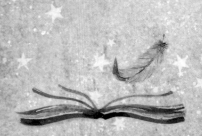

Famous Dreamers' Diaries

Have you ever been intrigued about the dreams of famous people? If so, you can read the oneiric visions of some who have shared their dreams in published works, whether it be in books solely dedicated to the subject or included in ones on a broader concept. These include:

William S. Burroughs, *My Education: A Book of Dreams*

Graham Greene, *A World of My Own: A Dream Diary*

Henry Rollins, *61 Dreams* (part of *Black Coffee Blues*)

Federico Fellini, *The Book of Dreams*

Jack Kerouac, *Book of Dreams*

Vladimir Nabokov, *Insomniac Dreams*

Table of Contents

PAGE	DATE	TITLE

Table of Contents

PAGE	DATE	TITLE

Crow

PAGE	THEMES	EVENING THOUGHTS
4	Falling	Work/Boss
20	Fear	Family Matters
26	Cooking	Work/Co-worker
28	Elevators	Elevators
34	Traffic	Work
52	Climbing	Project Deadline

PAGE:

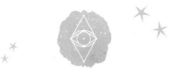

CHAPTER FIFTEEN

DECODING YOUR DREAMS

As you've likely experienced, the process of recalling, recording, and journaling your dreams itself can help to lift the veil that may have obscured your understanding as to what meaning they carried. Additionally, there are other approaches that can further help us decipher their significance. Of course, while working with a trained psychotherapist or dreamworker can offer you a personalized way to render more clarity, there are other ways that you can decode your dreams on your own, or with a community of others also interested in illuminating the wisdom of their oneiric visions. In this chapter, we'll explore approaches that will further help us to understand our dreams. We'll survey dream dictionaries, a Jungian technique known as Active Imagination, and popular divining methods. We'll also consider ways to tap into the power that comes through banding together with others, including working with a dreamwork partner and becoming involved with a dream group.

Dream Dictionaries and Symbol Books

One of the ways that many people gain insights into their dreams is by consulting a dream dictionary. As shared in the Introduction, interpretations of dream symbols were included in cuneiform tablets of the Library of Ashurbaniplal, dating from the seventh century BCE. While it was Artemidorus who is credited with writing one of the first and most comprehensive dream guide books back in the second century CE, his is not necessarily the oldest. Generally, dream dictionaries are books — or online databases — that are arranged in an A to Z format. You use them to look up an image that appeared in your dream to find out what it's commonly thought to represent. As you look through the interpretations, you may become more clear as to the potential meaning that the dream symbol possibly holds for you.

However, while these guides may help to catalyze your ability to become more fluent with images and their range of significance, it's important to not just adopt a particular meaning that's in the book and definitively apply it to your dream. Rather, it's important to see whether any of the associated meanings intuitively resonate with you and feel personally relevant. After all, while there are aspects of symbols that are thought to be universal, what one signifies to you may be different than what it does for another person. Sages throughout time, including Artemidorus himself, believed that the meaning of oneiric images was personal to the dreamer.

If reading about the different meanings of images is helpful to you in understanding your oneiric visions, there are other books that you can consult in addition to traditional dream dictionaries. These include books that catalog symbols that have held meaning for cultures throughout history. With their glossary-like approach, they may be similar to dream dictionaries, but not named as such. Again, though, be cautious in taking what is written and applying it to your dream without running it through your inner sense of truth to determine its personal veracity.

Active Imagination

Among his other breakthrough theories and accomplishments, Carl Jung pioneered a technique called Active Imagination, which can be used to bring forth a deeper level of understanding as to the insights that our dreams are dispatching. Active Imagination is a process by which you marry your conscious and unconscious minds to bring forth awareness and healing. And while it can be used as a general meditative and illuminative technique, it can also play a key role in helping us give voice to the wisdom that is carried forth by dream images and characters. When you use Active Imagination with your dreams, you begin by first finding yourself in a tranquil and reflective state. You invite in the recollections of a current dream, with the intention of having a dialogue with a character or symbol that it featured.

Once one of them emerges in your mind, you begin to converse with it. The trick is that you don't forcibly create the questions or answers, but rather allow them to arise, seeing what is stirred up and inspired by your imaginal mind. You beckon the dream image or character to provide you with clarification, asking them what they signified and what lessons they have for you. You can do Active Imagination quietly in your mind or in conversations out loud (and record them if you want). It can also be done with automatic writing, or through drawing, painting, music, or dance.

Doing Active Imagination with dreams can be quite an amazing process. You may find that it yields powerful surprises as you witness what spontaneously comes forth. After practicing it, especially with images or figures that have played a recurring starring role in your dreams, you may notice that they no longer appear with such frequency; the process of Active Imagination may allow you to get a direct line as to the communiqué they were carrying, making their role in your dreams no longer necessary. For many, it's best to start doing Active Imagination with someone trained in the method, such as a Jungian analyst or a professional schooled in the technique. Given that it gives your imaginal realm great freedom to express itself, it's thought that those who readily get lost in fantasy may want to exhibit caution in doing this practice, or only do it with a trained practitioner.

Tarot

If you work with tarot cards, you can turn to them to access more insights into what your dream may be revealing to you. If we think about how tarot cards are filled with images, reflect a visual landscape, and are embedded with archetypal symbols, it makes sense that they can help us garner more awareness as to what our dreams may be illuminating. Working with the tarot may aid you in accessing the part of your mind that is at home in this realm, acting as a conduit to help you better recall and understand your dreams.

There are several ways that you can work with the tarot to help decipher your dreams. One simple way is to think about a particular image that arose, about which you don't feel clear. Holding it in your mind's eye, pick a card and see what it reflects back to you. Another way is to do a tarot layout, as described on page 174.

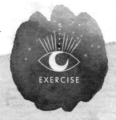

Deciphering Dreams with Tarot

To get more detailed insights into your dream, you can do a layout using three tarot cards. With this approach, it may be easier to work with the twenty-two cards of the Major Arcana, rather than the full deck.

1 Pick three cards, laying them down on a table in front of you from left to right.

2 Looking at the first card, consider that it represents the potential opportunity the dream (or a particular dream image) is pointing you toward. Reading about the card in a book, or looking to what you already know about it, see what it reflects to you about your dream.

3 Looking at the second card, consider that it represents a potential challenge about which the dream (or dream image) is making you aware. Reflect upon what this may signify.

4 Looking at the third card, consider that it is offering you guidance on how to orient to a situation in your life given what the first and second cards revealed. Reflect upon what this may signify.

If you have an ongoing tarot practice, you could also do more elaborate layouts — such as the Celtic Cross — using the whole deck to get even more detailed insights.

THE MAJOR ARCANA CARDS OF THE TAROT

While there are numerous tarot resources, both in print and online, for ready access, here is a list of the twenty-two Major Arcana cards, their associated number, and some keywords accorded with each.

0 – The Fool
Courage, innocence, freedom, risk-taking, rebellion, breakthroughs

1 – The Magician
Beginnings, learning, discipline, manifestation, intentions, communication

2 – The High Priestess
Intuition, reflection, contemplation, knowing, sacred knowledge, divine feminine

3 – The Empress
Love, pleasure, beauty, creativity, luxury, sensuality

4 – The Emperor
Authority, foundations, empowerment, responsibility, leadership, dignity

5 – The Hierophant
Tradition, community, faith, teacher, knowledge, sacred vows

6 – The Lovers
Discernment, choice, relationship crossroads, commitment, learning, wholeness

7 – The Chariot
Ambition, intuition, forward movement, self-realization, beginnings, integrity

8 – Strength
Patience, passion, self-love, gentleness, vulnerability, self-care

9 – The Hermit
Solitude, faith, inner journey, service, guidance, vigilance

10 – Wheel of Fortune
Change, opportunity, expansion, luck, new possibilities, flexibility

11 – Justice
Balance, harmony, adjustment, inner peace, truth, judgment

12 – The Hanged Man
Surrender, disillusionment, paradox, martyrdom, perspective, divinity

13 – Death
Endings, completion, transformation, liberation, internal change, regeneration

14 – Temperance

Art, learning, alchemy, creativity, integration, balance of opposites

15 – The Devil

Fear, obsession, control, power struggles, creativity, dark side

16 – The Tower

Fundamental change, destruction, chaos, dismantling, endings, healing

17 – The Star

Inspiration, destiny, imagination, dreams, creativity, future

18 – The Moon

Shadow, past, illusions, dreamscapes, deception, illumination

19 – The Sun

Freedom, innocence, new beginnings, enthusiasm, vitality, success

20 – Judgment

Accountability, reckoning, life review, truth, awakening, self-acceptance

21 – The World

Completion, empowerment, achievement, manifestation, big picture, leadership

Pendulum

Another way to gain insight into your dreams is by dowsing with a pendulum. The use of finding hidden information or items with this approach goes back thousands of years, with ancient Egyptian bas reliefs showing people using these instruments. A pendulum is composed of a string, usually a light chain, that has a weighted stone or crystal attached to it. It's designed in such a way that when held, the crystal or stone is able to swing in an unobstructed manner.

You can use a pendulum to access answers to questions, with certain observed movements signifying a specific answer and others a different one; generally, when using a pendulum, most people assign a certain movement to accord to a Yes response, another to a No response, and another to reflect a response that indicates uncertainty. People use pendulums for insights on a variety of subjects, including to probe more deeply into what their dreams may have signified.

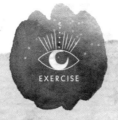

Using a Pendulum

If you're not clear about what a dream symbol means, you can see what insights you can access using the pendulum. Here's a simple way to do it:

1 Look in a dream dictionary or symbol book for all the meanings associated with the image in which you're interested in decoding.

2 Focusing upon one meaning at a time, as you're holding the pendulum, pose the question, "Is this what the dream image signifies for me?"

3 As you go through each possible meaning, see for which one/s the pendulum's movement yields an affirmative answer. This may help you refine your understanding as to the significance that your dream symbol contained.

The *I Ching*

The *I Ching* is a time-honored book that offers a wellspring of wisdom from Taoism and Confucianism. It features an oracular method to tap into prized philosophical knowledge, including to access more insights into your dreams. For over three thousand years, it's been used to provide guidance and counsel to people from all swaths of life, from kings to commoners. The *I Ching* is also known as *The Book of Changes*. It contains sixty-four hexagram designs, each of which has a name and number, and is associated with a trove of

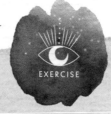

EXERCISE

Working with the I Ching

1   Focus on a question that you have about an aspect of your dream or its meaning in toto.

2   As you are doing this, toss your divination objects — whether yarrow sticks, coins, or specialized dice — onto a surface in front of you.

3   Consulting an *I Ching* book, determine which hexagram is mirrored by the result of your toss.

4   Read the resultant hexagram through the lens of answering your dream-meaning inquiry.

time-honored wisdom. To "consult the *I Ching*" — and discover the hexagram that mirrors your inquiry — you use a technique that involves throwing either yarrow sticks, coins, or specialized dice, and doing a calculation based upon what results.

Dreamwork Partners

One way to further understand what your dreams may be revealing is to work with a dreamwork partner. This would be someone that you trust, perhaps a relied-upon friend or colleague, who is also interested in dreamwork. They would need to be someone with whom you feel comfortable sharing the intimacies of your inner self, as revealed by what comes forth in your dreams.

Working with a dreamwork partner can not only help you to access deeper awareness as to what your dreams signify, but it will also assist you to more readily remember your dreams. After all, if you're committing to another person that you will be capturing and recounting your dreams, you will be motivated to do so. Doing dreamwork with a partner is a powerful way to not only dive deeper into your dreams, but it can help you to establish the strong relationship bond that comes from honestly sharing yourself with another person. Once you and your partner have decided that you would like to support each other in your dreamwork, set a few guidelines for engagement. Here are several steps to follow that will help you create a partnership that will be rewarding.

MAKE A TIME COMMITMENT

Decide upon a time frame, perhaps a month or two, to which you will commit to being dreamwork partners, after which time you can reevaluate how the process is serving you both. Knowing that your commitment is bounded and won't go on for an undetermined time, it will help each of you be more steadfast in your allegiance to the process.

DETERMINE YOUR SHARING FREQUENCY

Choose a consistent frequency with which to share your dreams with each other. Generally, anywhere from daily to weekly works best. If you're only sharing select dreams, you could even extend it to every other week. Beyond that, too much time passes, and the strength of the work seems to dissipate.

WAYS TO SHARE YOUR DREAMS

Determine how you want to share your dreams. Will you do so via email or video chat, on the phone or in person? You may also decide that you want to do some sort of hybrid approach if that works better for you. For some people, just having another person hear their dreams provides enough value. It enables them to feel witnessed, and the accountability of having to share dreams on a regular basis motivates them to focus on recording them. For others, however, the richness of the experience comes through getting their partner's reflections on their dreams, as that serves as a vehicle to help further discover their meanings.

HOW TO OFFER REFLECTIONS

If you decide to offer reflections upon each other's dreams, decide what type and how much you want. Is a sentence or two adequate, or do you both want what you receive to be more in-depth if the dream warrants it? Will you offer your thoughts on all the dreams that you each send to the other, or only on a select number? If the latter, decide who — the dreamer or their partner — gets to determine which dreams will get more in-depth treatment. Again, having these clear expectations as to what you give and what you receive does wonders for the relationship and the communication that it entails.

When giving reflection, it's a good practice to start with "If this were my dream …" It creates a boundary and clarifies that each of you is offering your personal associations, rather than stating an objective analysis of the dream. It reminds each person that it is truly the dreamer who has ownership over the dream, and, as such, is the one who knows what it really signifies. The other person is just offering perspectives that may help the dreamer realize what that significance is.

Dream Groups

While working with a dreamwork partner can help you access insights that may not otherwise be available, so can being part of a dream group. Also referred to as dream clubs, they offer a collective approach to mining the messages that may be carried in our dreams. One of the pioneers of the dream group model was Montague Ullman, MD (who, you may remember from chapter 7, was also a trailblazer in researching precognitive and telepathic dreams). What follows is a process you can use to coordinate a dream group meeting, which reflects many of the tenets that Ullman designed and tested over the years. The benefits of this approach are multi-fold, including having a group of people hold space for someone to share a dream elevates its significance. And, committing to an ongoing dreamwork practice can enhance participants' dream recall. Additionally, having numerous people offer their vantage points helps to further reveal the essence of the dreams shared. Plus, being part of a dream group can be a fun activity as it brings you together in a newly forged community, enjoying all the advantages that this yields.

Dream groups may be led by psychotherapists or dreamworkers, although just as likely they may be a group of laypersons who come together to share their collective interest. They may be in-person groups or those that meet online. If you can't find one, or don't align with any that exist, consider starting one. Put out an invitation to friends and colleagues who may be interested. You want the group to be small enough so that everyone can share, but large enough so that there is adequate heterogeneity and fodder for conversation. Many suggest that six to eight people is a good size.

Dream groups often meet weekly or biweekly. In the beginning, you may want to define a finite time frame for the group, perhaps getting everyone to commit to several months. After that, you can then reassess whether to extend it. And while the members may change, many dream groups find that they go on for years. To create a safe and reliable container for the dream group, it's good to have a few guidelines in place. These can include:

- Group members should speak about dreams with reverent appreciation and maintain a strong respect for one another.

- The group should adopt a stance of confidentiality. Nothing that is shared within the group should be discussed with anyone outside of it, and no recording should be allowed unless everyone in the group agrees. The exception to this could be that each member can share a dream of theirs that the group workshopped — and what they learned — with a friend or their therapist, but it should be done in a manner that safeguards the other members' privacy.

- Everyone should remember that the person who shares their dream is the ultimate authority on it. While others play an active role in its deciphering by giving reflection and asking questions that help the interpretation to unfold, ultimately it's the dreamer who knows the meaning it holds for them. The group just helps them discover it, acting as sherpas, supporting them on the journey to clarify the gift that it offers.

- The person who shares their dream gets to be in charge of declaring when they feel that the process of inquiry is complete for them, calling for the end of it. Even if others still believe there is more matter to be mined, the dreamer has the ultimate say on when they feel complete.

- Someone should assume the role of being the group leader. If it works for the group dynamic, you can change who assumes this role in subsequent gatherings. The leader shepherds the movement between the different stages of the process and keeps the conversation flowing.

STAGE 1: THE DREAMER SHARES

One person (or two, depending upon time) elects to share a dream that they found to be interesting, curious, and/or meaningful. It should be a dream that is recent enough so that they can remember its details, as well as what was transpiring in their life around the time that they had it. That said, if a group member has a dream from years ago that's stayed with them, and which they regard as important and impactful, they can share it. They should communicate as much of the dream as they remember and as much as they feel comfortable sharing. They should recount it without any editing or commentary, either about the dream or their waking life. It's important that they don't share any potential analysis, as they don't want to bias the group as to what their interpretation will be.

The group should listen intently and take notes if they desire. Some groups like to have the dreamer type up the dream, read it aloud, and then share a copy with everyone. This can be helpful in capturing details that may be otherwise missed while listening to the dream's retelling. After the dreamer shares their dream, members of the group can ask questions if they need clarification. These questions should be focused on the content of the dream, not what it may mean.

STAGE 2: THE GROUP MEMBERS SHARE

Next, the group members mirror back reflections to the dreamer. They share how the dream made them feel, what was stirred for them while listening to it. They should work with the images, seeing what arises for them in terms of metaphorical meanings. This can be done in a certain order; for example, by going around in a circle. Or the group members can share in a more spontaneous fashion.

As previously noted in the dreamwork partner section, it's always important for someone who is witnessing another's dream to have their reflections begin with the statement, "If this were my dream…" This helps to remind everyone that the only person who truly knows what the dream signifies is the person to whom it belongs, allowing them to maintain ownership of it. Members share reflections until the process feels complete; this is something that the leader can help distinguish.

If it feels right, someone can write down the group's reflections on a blackboard, whiteboard, or large notepad on an easel. This can be helpful, since it's often a good idea to synthesize what the group had shared before this step is complete. During this whole process, the dreamer remains silent, attentively listening.

STAGE 3: THE DREAMER AND THE GROUP DIALOGUE

In this stage, the dreamer notes which group members' reflections most notably resonated with them, and which ones didn't. To get deeper into the potential that this stage holds, the group can ask further questions of the dreamer: about their experience of the dream and how they feel it may relate to situations in their current life.

If a group member perceives that the dreamer isn't readily making connections between the dream and situations that are unfolding in their life, they can gently and compassionately nudge them by asking about what occurred the day before the dream. They can even inquire as to what they were thinking about before they went to bed. Yet, they shouldn't push the dreamer to make realizations that they are not ready to.

At some point, it becomes apparent when the process is finished and all that is to be evidenced has been brought forth. At this point, the leader can ask the group member who shared their dream if they feel that the group work is complete. If the dreamer has typed up and shared their dream, someone can read it aloud at the end, marking the closure of the process.

CHAPTER SIXTEEN

ASTRODREAMWORK

If you're looking for another way to work with your oneiric visions, consider using an astrological approach to dreaming, a method I call AstroDreamwork. Given that both dreams and astrology are vehicles for self-awareness, they can work together to synergistically help us access an even deeper level of understanding. As you'll see, astrology can aid us in accessing and translating the meaning of our dreams, while dreams give us insights that can further reveal the fount of self-knowledge potentiated within our astrology charts and the current zeitgeist through which we are living. Even if you don't know much about astrology, you may find that AstroDreamwork offers you supernal benefits.

A Traditional Practice

Astrology is a sacred art that has guided cultures throughout history. With roots dating back to Babylonia in the second millennium BCE, astrology has been used for providing counsel and guidance ever since. While it previously was the provenance of priests, physicians, and court advisors, in the twentieth century, it became ever more accessible to laypersons with the publication of the first horoscope columns. Today, as we continue to seek self-knowledge as well as glean answers to larger universal questions, astrology has made further inroads into popular culture.

The connection between astrology and dreams has roots at least as far back as medieval times. It was during this period that court astrologers would serve as counsel for kings, providing them with divinatory insights that would guide their approach to affairs of state, including when to arrange meetings or whether to proceed with battles. Some of these prized insights would come through interpreting the dreams of the nobility, as their oneiric visions were viewed as being divinely informed.

Astrologers today who practice medieval-astrology techniques use these classic principles when working with the dreams of their clients. Some of the notable texts that feature guidelines for this practice include *The Book of Astronomy* by Guido Bonatti, who, in the thirteenth century, served as advisor to numerous leaders, including Holy Roman Emperor Frederick II. Another classic tome is the *Complete Book on the Judgment of the Stars* by Ali Ibn Abi al-Rijal, written in the eleventh century and translated into Latin four centuries later.

Using these techniques, astrologers create charts for the moment a client asks them a question about a dream they've had. From there, they use methods to first assess whether the dream has value in understanding a pressing situation. If the dream is found to hold insights, the astrologer then looks to the planets in certain areas of the astrology chart to try to understand the nature of the dream. They then do further analysis to see if and how what occurred in the dream is likely to manifest in waking life, partially assessed by looking at key features of the Moon in the astrology chart. While this particular approach takes skill and experience, you need not be a practicing astrologer to be able to turn to astrology to access more awareness about your dreams. Following are numerous ways in which you can practice AstroDreamwork.

Your Signs, Your Dreams

Your personal astrology chart holds the keys to understanding the unique signatures that make you who you are. Your astrology chart can help you decipher what your dreams are revealing, while your dreams can unlock the mysteries of your astrology chart. And while astrologers who practice AstroDreamwork may minister to their client's dreams through the lens of their full natal chart, even a cursory understanding of your personal astrology can give you stellar insights into deciphering your dreams. You only need to look to your Sun sign (what you answer when someone asks you, "What's your sign?"), and if you know them, your Moon and Ascendant signs as well. (Don't readily know your Moon and Ascendant signs? Check the Resources section on page 223 for a way to discover them.) As zodiacal signs express who we are, their characteristics are those that we tap into during our waking life. Knowing about our signs, we can see why it may be that we act a certain way, ruminate about a particular topic, approach situations through a particular emotional vantage point, or find ourselves motivated toward certain activities. These are facets of ourselves that also show up in our dreams.

On page 188, you'll find a list of the twelve zodiacal signs, as well as some characteristics and symbols associated with each. Since the sign that our Sun is in — as well as the ones that our Moon and Ascendant are in — represent core principles of who we are, we may find that their associated signatures appear in our dreams with some regularity. After all, they are reflections of the archetypes with which we are connected, and how we express much of who we are, whether in our waking life or our dreaming life.

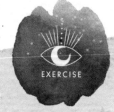

EXERCISE

A Stellar Approach to Dreams

Here's a simple AstroDreamwork approach you can try.

- Since most people know their Sun sign, first read the keywords associated with yours. Remember that the Sun represents your vitality, identity, and the things that have you shine. And so, if you notice a dream that is filled with many of these themes and symbols, it may be that you're working through issues related to further expressing your identity and what it is that truly makes you tick.

- Now look to your Moon sign. Because the Moon represents what we find nourishing, as well as our unconscious instincts, the sign that it is in gives us distinct insights into what our dreams may be revealing about how we orient emotionally. If archetypes related to your Moon sign are quite present in a dream, it may be that you're trying to work out some powerful emotional issues and/or gain insights into how you can take better care of yourself.

- After that, look to your Ascendant sign (also known as the Rising sign), which signals how we present ourselves and move through the world. It also represents how we perceive the external world and orient to it. As our dreams reflect the way that we navigate through life, their backdrops may be infused with telltale images associated with our Ascendant sign. If your dream is particularly flush with concepts related to it, it may be that you're trying to solve challenges related to how to maneuver a current situation and/or you're reconsidering the way you want to present your image to the world.

- If you don't already know them, you can find resources to discover your Moon and Ascendant signs on page 223.

THE ZODIAC SIGNS

Aries

Desire nature. Fast movements.
Battle of wills. Sharp objects. Impatience.
Warriors. Swords. Guns. Head. Rams.

Taurus

Sensual delights. Practical solutions.
Slow movements. Resistance to change.
Luxury items. Verdant scenery. Flowers.
Routines. Neck. Bulls.

Gemini

Dual approaches. Gathering information.
Need for variety. Intellectual orientation.
Schoolrooms. Breathing. Libraries.
Messengers. Arms. Twins.

Cancer

Family orientation. Maternal instincts.
Feeding people. Indirect movements.
Containers of safety. Kitchens. Gardens.
Moon. Stomach. Crabs.

Leo

Artistic expressions. Dramatic
performances. Romantic love. Pride.
Sun. Royalty. Gold. Children. Heart.
Lions.

Virgo

Filing systems. Fitness studios. Digestion.
Perfectionism. Crafts. Organization.
Details. Agriculture. Pets. Maidens.

Libra

Art galleries. Social gatherings.
Courtrooms. Equality. Indecision.
Diplomacy. Partnerships. Roses.
Skin. Scales.

Scorpio

Buried treasures. Deep emotions. Secrets.
Darkness. Transformation. Passion. Money.
Toilets. Genitals. Scorpions.

Sagittarius

Foreign lands. Religious sites. Big picture.
Truth. Philosophy. Adventures. Travel.
Liver. Archery. Horses.

Capricorn

Skeletal system. Old age. Time. Success.
Blueprints. Endurance. Delays. Knees.
Mountains. Goats.

Aquarius

Futuristic visions. Technological
advances. Humanitarian missions. Gadgets.
Innovation. Rebellions. Spaceships. Ankles.
Urns. Stars.

Pisces

Unconditional love. Blurred boundaries.
Mystical pursuits. Oceans. Sacrifices.
Compassion. Fog. Magic. Feet. Fish.

Dreams and the Moon

Throughout time, the Moon has represented our emotional nature, the sea of feelings in which we swim, and the tides of our personal unconscious. As such, it also is an archetypal symbol that represents our dreams. There are numerous ways that you can turn to the Moon when working with your oneiric visions.

THE LUNAR CYCLE

Throughout the month, the Moon moves through a cycle in which it appears to grow with light, reaching the culmination of a Full Moon. It then proceeds to have its illumination wane, receding back to darkness, before it again becomes a New Moon. The monthly New Moon is said to be a time in which we can initiate new beginnings. Several days before this new lunar cycle begins, the Moon holds and projects less and less — and finally an absence — of the Sun's rays. Referred to as the Balsamic Moon, this is the

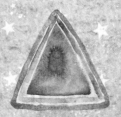

The Four Elements

Zodiacal signs are often grouped together based upon the element to which they belong. Here are some qualities and symbols associated with each. You may be able to get more insights into what your dream symbols are revealing by looking to see if those associated with the elements of your Sun, Moon, and Ascendant appear with frequency in your dreams.

Fire (Aries, Leo, Sagittarius)
Flames, spirited action, candles, vertical movements, red, orange

Earth (Taurus, Virgo, Capricorn)
The earth, practical matters, physical structures, sensual experiences, green, brown

Air (Gemini, Libra, Aquarius)
Communication, conversations, balloons, wind, horizontal movement, yellow

Water (Cancer, Scorpio, Pisces)
Water, the sea, faucets, boats, aquatic creatures, blue

phase of the lunar cycle in which we're oriented to letting go and finding direction through connecting to the depth of illumination within ourselves; it's a time to be still, meditative, and reflective, seeing what arises from the depths of our intuition. As such, it's also an especially gorgeous time to tune in to what's being revealed through our dreams.

Many people like to make New Moon intentions, planting seeds for what they want to usher in during the month-long lunar cycle. By doing dream incubation (which we explored in chapter 11) in the last days of the Balsamic Moon and first days of the New Moon phases, we can gain further clarity as to what we may want to hone our focus upon to manifest over the coming four weeks. Before going to bed, ask that your dreams contain directionality as to what is ripe for growth in the ensuing month. You could pose this as a general inquiry, asking yourself something like, "Dreams, please point me to an understanding of what intention I should make for this new month."

Or, if you want to further target this practice, you can work with the energy of the sign in which the New Moon will appear. For example, for the New Moon that occurs during Capricorn season (the third week of December to the third week of January), you could ask your dreams to share insights with you into objectives you can undertake related to how to be more productive or efficient. Or, during the New Moon that takes place during Leo season (the third week of July through the third week of August), you could request clues as to how to bring more joy and creativity into your life. Look to page 188 to gain more insights into what each of the signs represents and therefore what a focused New Moon dream practice could target. You can find a way to discover dates for the New Moons in the Resources section on page 223. Additionally, if you know your birth chart, you can get more details into what each New Moon is inspiring for you personally. For example, if it connects with your Venus, the following weeks may bring lessons in love, while if it takes up residency in the 11th House of your astrology chart, the coming month may hold opportunities for community work. Knowing this, you can then refine your dream-incubation inquiry.

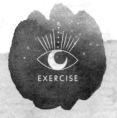

Full Moon Dreams

The days around the monthly Full Moon seem as if they are filled with heightened energy. While some people find that they are more likely to have disrupted sleep during this period, others note that their dreams are more vivid and active around the time of the Full Moon. Be aware of any sleep and dream patterns that arise for you during this lunation.

1   Pay attention each month to when the Full Moon occurs.

2   Keep track of it in your dream journal, making a notation on the days that it takes place.

3   See whether the dreams you have around the Full Moon have a different level of intensity or feature certain themes. Note whether your sleeping pattern has a unique quality during this time of the month.

4   After a few months of tracking this, look through your dream journal to see if you can identify any patterns that connect your Full Moon dreams.

191

ECLIPSES

Each year, between four and seven eclipses occur. Some accord with New Moons (solar eclipses) and some with Full Moons (lunar eclipses). Even if we can't see an eclipse in the sky where we live, these celestial events are thought to coincide with powerful, life-changing events and reflections. Mark the eclipses on your calendar, and then see if your dreams have a different tone or yield unique perspectives the week before and after them. Once again, if you know your birth chart, you may be able to generate additional insights, since you will know which realms of your life the eclipses are highlighting.

Mercury, Venus, and Mars Retrograde

When it comes to astrological awareness, one of the phenomena that continues to capture many people's attention is Mercury Retrograde. As it turns out, the retrograde cycle of this quicksilver messenger planet — plus those of Venus and Mars — can be a time when doing AstroDreamwork can be very fruitful. To understand why, let's start with defining what it means when a planet is in its retrograde cycle. When this occurs, the planet appears — from our vantage point on Earth — to be moving backward in the sky, in motion apparently distinct from that of other celestial bodies. And while the perceived shift is an illusion caused by the paced pathways in which the different planets, including the Earth, orbit the Sun, astrologically, the retrograde cycle of planets is accorded with special meaning.

As the planets revisit territory already traveled during their retrograde phase, we are encouraged to do the same, going back to the past with fresh eyes. Our waking thoughts may feature our retracing of situations that we've already traversed...and so may what arises in our dreams. During these planetary retrogrades, you may notice more emphasis on people, places, situations, objects, and ideas from the past in your dreams. And as we reencounter previously traveled landscapes, we may see how our dreams are helping us to craft understanding in our present, based upon further acceptance and awareness of what came before, so that we can move forward with more clarity. And while, from our perspective on Earth, all planets experience a retrograde cycle, those of the trio known as the personal planets — Mercury, Venus, and Mars — seem to be a time when we access insights that inform us on a more individual level. As such, they serve as a stellar focus for AstroDreamwork.

MERCURY RETROGRADE

Mercury is the planet of communication. During its thrice-yearly retrograde cycle, we revisit ideas from the past in order to gain a new perspective, one that can bolster our ability to more clearly share thoughts and move about in the world. To this aim, during its retrograde cycle, symbols of Mercury — such as books, mail, cars, bicycles, planes, computers, and bridges — may populate our dreams. See what they are reflecting to you about learning and communicating from a different angle.

VENUS RETROGRADE

Venus Retrograde occurs every eighteen months, and is a time period in which we reevaluate what we value. During it, we may also find ourselves reconsidering our relationship realm and our approach to partnerships. In the course of its retrograde, symbols of Venus — such as luxury items, money, mirrors, lovers, objects of beauty, cosmetics, and artwork — may appear in our dreams. See how they point you toward further understanding the ways in which you can infuse your life with more worth and richness.

MARS RETROGRADE

Occurring every two-plus years, Mars Retrograde is a stretch of time during which we may find ourselves further understanding just what it is that we desire, as well as how we design the strategies with which we pursue what we covet. It's also a time to gather more understanding about our relationship with anger and frustration. During Mars Retrograde, symbols of this planet — such as swords, knives, fire, battles, warriors, athletes, sexual pursuits, and the color red — may appear more frequently in our dreams. See how they may aim your attention toward the ways in which you're reconsidering how you cultivate and direct your energy and will.

Remember to pay special attention to images or scenes that involve reflections of the past during all the retrograde cycles. Also note that it's often the days around the beginning and ending of these periods in which the themes associated with these planets, and the awareness we're encouraged to discover, may be more concentrated. Consider paying special attention to your dreams during these nights. Find a way to learn the dates for upcoming retrograde cycles of Mercury, Venus, and Mars in the Resources section.

CHAPTER SEVENTEEN

NATURAL REMEDIES FOR DREAMING

In chapter 3, we explored natural remedies that could support relaxation and engender slumber. Let's now review those — including flower essences and crystals — that may help us further connect to our dreams. In this chapter, you'll also learn all about herbal dream pillows, including how to make your own.

Flower Essences

There are numerous ways in which flower essences can help to inspire our dreamwork. (For more on how to use flower essences, see page 49.)

Angelica

Angelica helps us to feel wrapped in protection in the liminal space of our dreams, more open to the spiritual guidance that can come forth. And with that, it may inspire a deeper experience of connection, attunement, and remembrance within our oneiric visions.

Cosmos

There are times when we can "see" our dreams upon waking, but it's hard to access them in a way that allows us to communicate them in words. Cosmos flower essence helps to bridge the third-eye and throat chakras, which may assist us in giving voice to our dreams and documenting them more readily.

Iris

If your dreams feel lifeless and less than animated, consider Iris flower essence. It is thought to add color, both literally and figuratively, to our visions, helping us to rekindle the creative inspiration that dreams can offer us.

Morning Glory

If you wake up with a dulled and drowsy feeling, as if part of you hasn't returned from your dreamscape, Morning Glory may be a great flower essence to use. It can help us ground back in our bodies and be more in sync with rhythms of light and dark, awake and sleep.

Mugwort

Mugwort is a plant traditionally associated with dreaming. In its flower essence form, it's said to stimulate the psyche's receptive capacity for awareness during our oneiric journeys. Additionally, it may help us to be better able to bridge awareness between dreams and waking life, enhancing the integrated weaving of insights experienced in each into the other.

Shasta Daisy

Sometimes we can understand parts of our dream, but we're unclear as to how they all weave together. To help forge a clearer vision as to the broader meaning of a dream and how all the pieces may thread together as a whole, try Shasta Daisy flower essence.

St. John's Wort

St. John's Wort was traditionally heralded as the flower of protection. In its essence form, it's thought to offer protection to those who are psychically sensitive and feel undefended in their dreams. Therefore, it may be a helpful remedy for people who experience nightmares.

Star Tulip

Star Tulip is a wonderful essence to help augment inner listening and receptivity. That makes it great for use in activities, such as dreaming, in which we want assistance tuning in to the awareness that's streaming forth from the depths of our minds.

Crystals

Many people like to incorporate crystals and gemstones into their self-care regimens, including using them for enhancing sleep and dreams. They are so beautiful that even those who don't accord them with wisdom significance find that there's something so alluring about them: the way they capture and reflect light, the dance of colors in which they are imbued, and the energy — sometimes subtle and sometimes powerful — that they emit. And that's not even considering the awe that arises when you stop to think how they are the result of thousands and thousands of years of geological transformation, fostering a feeling of connection to the Earth and a sense of timelessness.

And while some think of them as a new-age fad, the power accorded to them cuts across time and culture. It's been noted that the ancient Egyptians buried their dead with crystals, as they were thought to protect them in their journey to the afterlife. It's said that the first-century CE Roman general Plautius instructed his soldiers to cover themselves with hematite, found in the soil upon which they were fighting; it was thought that doing so would bestow upon them protection from Mars, the god of war, during the battles in which they were engaged. And let's not forget that in the *Vedas*, the classic Indian texts, there includes numerous mentions of the remedial effects of gemstones. Additionally, modern-day discoveries have found that some gemstones carry important properties. For example, certain quartz crystals have piezoelectricity, generating electrical potential when mechanical stress is applied to them.

CHOOSING DREAMWORK CRYSTALS

There are hundreds, if not thousands, of different types of crystals and gemstones; how do you choose which ones to weave into your dreamwork? Here are three different approaches that you can use.

1. Crystal Nature

The first approach is to explore crystals that have been noted to have properties that benefit different aspects of dreamwork. These include:

- *Enhance Dream Recall:* Celestite, Kyanite
- *Encourage Lucid Dreaming:* Danburite, Pink Moonstone

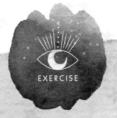

Working with Crystals

There are numerous ways that you can work with crystals to inspire your dreams. Some ideas include:

■ Use them as a talisman, placing them under your pillow, on your nightstand, or on your dream altar. Just knowing that your intentionally chosen gemstones are within view may help amplify your dream connection.

■ Lay out gemstones in a crystal grid to give more power to your dream intentions. You can find details on how to do this in books and online.

■ Crystal-grid your bedroom. For example, you could place a special crystal in each corner of the room. After doing so, use a wand-shaped crystal to connect the energetic matrix. Doing this could both amplify the energy of your bedroom sanctuary and make it feel more like a protected space.

■ As you incorporate crystals into your dreamwork practice, tune in to see what, if any, shifts emerge over the coming week or so. Do certain colors appear in your dreams? Specific themes? Particular feeling tones? Note this in your dream journal so that you can assess the effects of this practice.

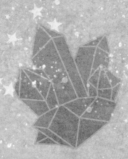

Crystals and Dream Incubation

Here are two ways to work with crystals and the dream-incubation practice that we explored in chapter 11. One simple way is to just hold your gemstone in your hand as you focus in on your incubation intention. Before you drift off to sleep, place it under your pillow, or on your nightstand. As you wake up, once again hold your crystal in your hand and see if it helps you further remember what came forth in your dream. Another technique is to have your crystal grid be focused upon your dream-incubation intention. Write down your intention on a piece of paper, fold it, and place that in the center of your crystal mandala. Design your grid around your intention, choosing a layout shape (i.e., spiral, infinity loop, etc.) that resonates with you, placing crystals in the various spots. Finally, place a center crystal on top of your written intention. Using a crystal wand, trace all of the crystals to unite them vibrationally. As you go to sleep, focus upon what insights you want your dream to reveal, holding the image of your crystal grid in your mind's eye.

- **Foster Understanding of a Dream's Meaning:** Amethyst, Selenite

- **Promote Dreams of Insight:** Jade, Moonstone

- **Help Protect Against Nightmares:** Pink Calcite, Smoky Quartz

2. Crystal Themes

In the second method, you choose crystals that are focused upon the themes that you're finding yourself to be working through in your dreams. While a crystal dictionary can help you find those supportive of an array of aims, here are a few examples to consider.

- **Bolstered Self-Esteem:** Citrine, Chrysoberyl

- **Enhanced Creativity:** Carnelian, Turquoise

- **Greater Self-Love and Compassion:** Rose Quartz, Rhodochrosite

- **Healing from Addictions:** Amethyst, Iolite

- **Working Through Relationship Challenges:** Dioptase, Lapis Lazuli

3. Crystal Curiosity

The third way to decide upon crystals to use in dreamwork is to be led by your intentional curiosity. Visit a gemstone store and see which ones call to you. Focus upon the benefit that you'd like the crystal to provide, whether that's helping you better remember your dreams, access more lucidity, feel more protected should you have a nightmare, or any of your other oneiric aims. Based upon this, see which ones you are magnetized toward.

Herbal Dream Pillows

As we saw in chapter 3, teas made from herbs have slumber-inspiring properties. Another way that you can use herbs and botanicals to support your sleep and dreams is by making a dream pillow. Also referred to as comfort pillows or dreamtime pillows, they have been used for centuries as part of nighttime rituals. One of the first recipes for dream pillows was included in the 1606 book *Ram's Little Dodeon: A Brief Epitome of the New Herbal, or History of Plants* by William Ram. It featured rose petals combined with mint powder and clove powder. Both King George III and Abraham Lincoln are said to be among those who used a pillow filled with hops to help them sleep.

How may they work? Fragrances connect to the brain's limbic system and help encourage different feeling states, including pacifity and relaxation. As such, the subtle scents emitted from a dream sachet tucked underneath your pillow, or placed on your nightstand, can help lull you to sleep and to dream. Their effects, though, may not cease once slumber falls upon you. After all, our brains are thought to process smells when we sleep, with researchers suggesting that fragrance experienced while dozing may impact the emotional currents of our dreams.

While premade dream pillows are available, it's also easy to make your own. It could be a fun and creative project to do solo or with friends or family. Also consider it as another DIY activity that you could do with your children or grandchildren if you're looking for an additional way to help them forge a connection with their dreams. (See the next page for tips on making your own herbal dream pillow.)

How to Make a Dream Pillow

A dream pillow consists of two parts: the covering, and the herbs that will fill it.

The Covering

You could go a very simple route and choose to use premade small cotton muslin bags with drawstrings. The advantage to this approach is that it cuts down on preparation time. The drawback is that it may not be as pretty and personalized. Or you could make your own pillow covering. To do so:

1   Buy natural fiber fabric such as cotton, linen, or silk. Wash it before creating your pillow covering so that any dyes or odors can be released.

2   Determine the size you want your finished pillow to be and cut it about ¾ to 1 inch (2 to 2.5 cm) bigger on all sides to allow for sewn seams. Some people prefer square ones while others like them rectangular. The only real confine you have is that it fits neatly under your pillow. If you like more fragrance, then use a larger size; if you'd rather it be subtler, opt for a smaller one.

3　Fold your fabric with the right sides facing each other. Sew it on the two sides perpendicular to the fold, as well as one-quarter of the way in on either side on the part that opposes the fold. Just make sure you leave enough room to put the herbs and flowers in.

4　Turn the pillowcase through the opening so that it is right side out.

5　Fill it with the herbs and flowers of your choice; you can either put them in loose or place them in a smaller muslin bag, and then fill the rest of the pillow with stuffing material.

6　Stitch up the opening. You can either do the whole project with a sewing machine or sew it by hand. If you'd rather not sew, you can always use seam tape, which just needs to be ironed to create closure.

The Herbs

There are numerous dried herbs and flowers you can use to fill your dream pillow. While the following are some of those traditionally used, if you have a favorite whose scent brings you joy, don't hesitate to include it. Just remember to briefly rub the dream pillow when you get into bed, as this will help to release its natural fragrances.

Lavender | With its sweetly floral scent, lavender is one of the premier flowers associated with calm and relaxation. Research has found that it helps increase levels of melatonin, the hormone necessary for good sleep. It also seems to have memory-boosting qualities, with one study suggesting that one of its chief constituents (linalool) could reduce the cognitive impairment that occurs with REM deprivation.

Mugwort | The Greek goddess Artemis, from which mugwort gets its botanical name (*Artemisia douglasiana*), was a Moon deity. When we remember that the Moon, archetypally, is associated with sleep and dreams, it's no coincidence that this is one of the herbs prized by a multitude of societies for its ability to herald vivid and prophetic dreams. Many native tribes, including the Paiute and Chumash (the latter who refer to mugwort as "dream sage"), use it to promote sacred dreaming.

Rose Petals | Take inspiration from *Ram's Little Dodeon* and include rose petals in your dream sachet (see page 199). The fragrance of rose is thought to be calming and reduce anxiety. Plus, it infuses one with a sense of romanticism and love, thoughts of which are lovely to fall asleep to, and which may inspire heart-opening dreamscapes.

Rosemary | Greek scholars wore wreathes of rosemary to abet their studying, as it was prized for aiding concentration and fortifying memory, qualities supported by many research studies. And while it brightens the mind, it does so while promoting relaxation. This makes it a great fragrance for not only galvanizing dreams, but also helping you remember them in the morning.

Yarrow | Yarrow flowers, with their fresh and herbaceous scent, can make a beautiful addition to a dream sachet. One of yarrow's reputed properties — its ability to energetically create a sheath of protection — is a plus for those who want to feel shielded during sleep. Plus, yarrow may also bring visions of love; in times past, young women would place yarrow beneath their pillow and say a little prayer in hopes of meeting their future husband in their dream.

Others | Hops are among the most traditionally used herbs for promoting sleep. Roman chamomile is relaxing and thought to protect against nightmares in folk medicine. Lemon balm is known for its calming properties. Orris root is added to dream pillows to extend the fragrance of the other flowers and herbs.

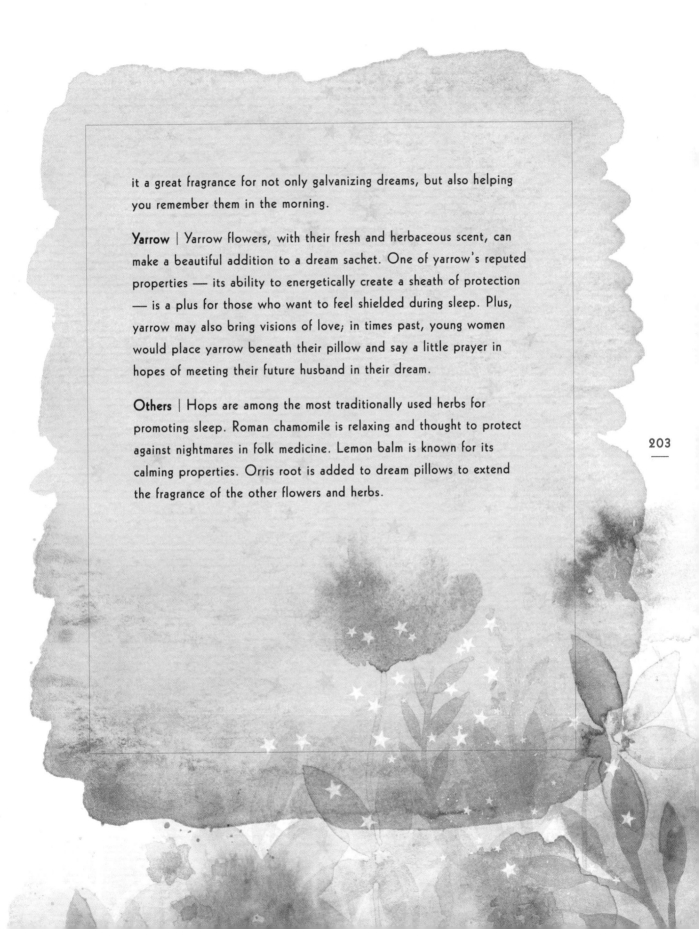

inspiring children's dreams

CHILDREN AND SLEEP

If we see dreams as a vehicle that brings us awareness and well-being, then helping children forge a relationship with them may be one of the greatest gifts we can give to our little ones. Traveling life with dreams as their companion can help enhance their self-awareness, assisting them in working through emotional issues, amplifying their creativity, and bolstering their problem-solving abilities. While regularly speaking with children about dreams may not be customary in our Western society, it is a commonplace activity in cultures around the world. Encouraging children to have a connection with their dreams is thought to be a way in which they can tap into their inner wisdom, guidance, and healing potential. Talking to your children about their dreams may be something you find to have many benefits, not only for them but also for your relationship. However, before we dive into how to help your children be inspired by their dreams (which we'll do in chapter 19), let's first explore something that's fundamental to their ability to dream well...helping them to sleep well.

Inspiring Sleep

As we know, sleep is elemental for good health, both physically and emotionally, no matter our age. And given sleep's essential function in growth and cognitive development, it's no surprise that we need more of it when we're young. Reflecting the National Sleep Foundation's recommendations, there's a significant difference between our needs and those of our children. Whether it's the 14 to 17 hours required by newborns or the 8 to 10 hours recommended for teenagers, or any of the ranges suggested for children in between, the amount of sleep kids should get is higher than the 7 to 9 hours that adults should.

Therefore, it's important to positively frame sleep for children. Encouraging them to revere sleep at an earlier age can help set them up for success in later life. Plus, their getting

205

adequate sleep can provide a spectrum of benefits for them in the here and now; it inspires proper growth and development, it encourages good mood and emotional resilience, and it can help them flourish in school. Regarding the last benefit, to understand the advantage that good sleep yields, we need only look at research that shows that children with sleep deficits demonstrate impaired attention, reduced motivation to learn, and encumbered academic achievement. And, of course, their getting good sleep is integral to connecting to the richness of their dreams. One way to encourage children's sleep is through having them partake in bedtime rituals.

Bedtime Rituals

Most kids love rituals. They help them feel safe and secure. Plus, they are an activity that you can share. Having children feel calm before they sleep goes a long way in helping them have a good night's sleep, perhaps even reducing their proclivity for nightmares. Some of the rituals below may be better suited for kids of certain ages than others. Some can be done together, while others are those you can encourage your child to do on their own. And while your teenager may not want you involved in their pre-sleep activities, sharing with them how certain routines can enhance their sleep and dreams may have them be curious enough to explore them on their own.

RECOUNTING THE DAY

If you haven't already had dedicated one-on-one time earlier in the evening, take the opportunity to have your child share about their day. Have them see this as a way to say farewell to their today as they open up to sleep and dreams, and then to their tomorrow. Consider having them tell you at least one thing that they worried about during the day and one thing for which they were grateful.

PRACTICING A SHORT MEDITATION

If your child needs more encouragement to wind down, you could do a short meditation practice with them. Have them choose a word that they like and focus upon it as they breathe in and breathe out. They can either keep their eyes open or shut. Alternatively, you could lead them through a shortened version of a progressive muscle relaxation exercise (see page 41) to help them further unwind their mind and their body.

LULLING THEM TO SLEEP

Originally used as a vehicle to pass down wisdom to children, lullabies — with their rocking rhythm — are a soothing sleep aid. If your child is too old for a lullaby, play some relaxing music. Remember that the light from tech devices, let alone the animating content, may inhibit slumber; thus, try to have them avoid screen time a couple of hours before sleep.

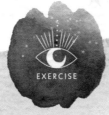

EXERCISE

Relaxing Breathwork

Help center your child by having them do simple breathing exercises for a few minutes. Instead of their doing the breathwork practices that you may do, it's better for them to do child-geared ones, since kids breathe at different rates than adults.

1 Have them inhale through their nose and exhale through their mouth with pursed lips.

2 Encourage them to breathe slowly into their diaphragm, placing a hand or a stuffed animal on their belly so that they can see it go up and down.

3 Have them do this for several minutes or until they feel more centered and calmer.

CREATING PERSONALIZED RITUALS

There may be other things that would help your child be more able to settle down into sleep. Ask them what they would like. Perhaps it's arranging their stuffed animals in a certain way, saying a prayer, being told a story, or something else.

Your Child's Bedroom

Paying special attention to our bedroom, having it be as comfortable and healthful as it can be, can go a long way in inspiring us to sleep and dream better. Many of the tips in chapter 4 can be applied to your child's bedroom. Additionally, involving your children in decorating or arranging their bedroom can invoke a greater sense of agency within them and have them feel more comfortable in their space. This can help them feel more settled when embarking upon sleep and dreams.

Of course, their involvement should be age-appropriate, with older kids having more choice than younger children. However, even little ones can be consulted when it comes to certain decisions, whether it be where to put their favorite stuffed animal or what color they want their bedsheets to be. If your children share a bedroom, make sure both feel that there are areas in the space that mirror comfort to them and reflect their individuality.

Allocate an area for them to keep their dream journal. If your teenage kids are exploring ways to connect with and work with their dreams, tell them about dream altars (see page 56). Have them pick out a dreamcatcher to hang in their bedroom; or consider making one together, as it can be a fun craft project. All of this can help your children feel that their bedrooms are a safe space that is nurturing and to which they can retreat. Not only will this help to engender their ability for self-soothing, but it will also help them to further align with their sleep, and their dreams.

DREAMCATCHERS

As a way to have your child connect to their dreams more and feel protected should they have nightmares, consider hanging a dreamcatcher above their bed. Talismanic items thought to have originated in the culture of the native Ojibwe peoples, dreamcatchers were designed to protect young children from bad dreams. Legend notes that originally Asibikaashi (Spider Women) would weave a web of protection for sleeping children.

Mothers and grandmothers followed in her tradition, creating these protective charms to safeguard their young.

Part of the beauty that the dreamcatcher may provide for your child is the story of its origin. It can help them connect to yet another tradition, as well as understand the universality of the dream experience. It's also important because, like with anything that originates in a culture that is not our own, it is always good practice to know from where something emerged, the meaning behind it, and the reverence with which it was treated.

Dreamcatchers feature a center hoop usually made from willow wood, with sinew or fiber strung through it to create a web design that features a central opening. Bad dreams are thought to get stuck in the web while good ones can pass through the dreamcatcher. It may also have feathers or beads hanging down, upon which the good dreams descend from the web and then fall upon the child sleeping below. If you buy a dreamcatcher, consider getting one that was handmade by a native craftsperson. Or buy the materials and make one with your child, as this can be yet another way to involve them in a dream-enriching experience.

Folkoric Characters

Legends throughout different cultures feature characters that help connect children to sleep and dreams. These include:

Baku

Baku is a mythical creature that children in Japan call out to after having a nightmare in hopes that it will devour their bad dreams.

La Dormette

A French sleep fairy who wanders around as night falls and sprinkles sand into the eyes of children, La Dormette is said to help little ones fall asleep and have pleasant dreams.

Sandman

Appearing in Scandinavian folktales, the Sandman lulls children to sleep and helps bring on their dreams by sprinkling sand or dust in their eyes.

Wee Willie Winkle

A character in a Scottish nursery rhyme, Wee Willie Winkle — who runs through the town in his nightgown checking on whether kids are asleep — has come to be a personification of slumber for many.

CHAPTER NINETEEN

CHILDREN AND DREAMS

Having dreams be a topic of conversation can help your kids see them as a source of inspiration, a way to gain more awareness about challenges facing them, and a wellspring for their creative development. Instead of feeling ashamed or hiding the feelings that emerge in their dreams, knowing that dreams are normal and being able to share them with someone without judgment can be exceptionally powerful. And if they have nightmares or dreams that disturb them, knowing that someone will listen to them can be soothing and comforting.

Given that children are less socially filtered than adults, their imaginations are stronger, and it's such a gift to help encourage it to flourish. Tapping into the language of dreams can do this. Additionally, connecting with your children about dreams will also foster your relationship; it's an amazing opportunity to know your child better and another way for them to see you as being encouraging and supportive. Dreams can be fodder not only for family conversations, but also shared creative endeavors. And while helping them understand what their dreams may be reflecting is valuable, the virtues of this practice exceed that. Even just having your child give voice to their dreams, and having them see that you are listening to them and appreciating the unique experience that they had, can itself provide exceptional benefit. As you'll see, this chapter describes many ways to help your children forge a connection with their dreams, as well as ways to work with them. Remember, though, this isn't an all-or-nothing pursuit. You may find that even just occasionally asking them about their dreams can open up a whole new world, for themselves and in your relationship with them.

Dreaming with Children

On some level, children's dreams are like ours. Some are good dreams and others may be nightmares. Some may have them emotionally processing feelings, while others may be a replay of mundane events. And they, like us, may also have big dreams, those filled with archetypal concepts, the knowledge of which seems to go beyond their years. Regardless of the type of dreams they have, here are ways that you can connect with your kids about them.

INSPIRE THEIR CURIOSITY

Talk about the power of dreams, and how they can be helpful in feeling happier and more confident in their lives. Tell them about famous people whose dreams preceded their inventing great things or creating masterful pieces of art (see page 16 for ideas). Share with them how some of the most popular kids' books — some that may even be their favorites — have dreams as a starring role (see page 213 for ideas).

DIALOGUE ABOUT THEIR DREAMS

For some kids, just acknowledging that they had a dream that they remembered is fulfilling enough. For others, though, discussing them may be something that

Benefits of Discussing Dreams with Children

- Has them realize dreams are a normal part of life

- Forges a connection of trust within the family

- Allows you to know each other better

- Creates another outlet for creativity

- Helps them develop new skills

- Offers a way to work through emotional challenges

- Makes them feel seen and heard

- Provides them the space to give voice to current concerns

- Stretches their minds, helping them see things from new angles

- Supports them in dealing with their fears

- Forms the basis for a new family activity

- Inspires their imagination

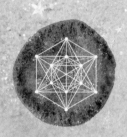

Characteristics of Children's Dreams

Children's dreams reflect their developmental stage, as well as the concerns that they face in their waking life. The structure and content of their dreams evolve as they get older. Perhaps because they are dealing with more unknowns and exploring ways to master the multitude of new experiences that they face, children have nightmares more frequently than adults. For more on the characteristics of children's dreams, see chapter 6.

they find fun and helpful. There are many ways to approach a dream, many paths through which you can invite them to share their dream and connect with it. Below you'll find some possible suggestions. Remember that there is no strict formula to follow per se: certain children may align better with certain questions and different ways that a dream inquiry may be sequenced and paced. Just make sure to customize the questions to reflect your communication styles.

How was your dream?

This is often a good entry approach, as it's open-ended and neutral, allowing your child to answer in a host of different ways. Even if their response is a simple good, boring, scary, exciting, okay, or another one-word answer, you'll get immediate insight into their top-line perspective on it. You also then have the beginning of a lexicon — their own — with which you can mirror back to them and further inquire about their dream. Of course, for some kids, rather than yielding just a one- or two-word answer, the "How was your dream?" question may produce a whole treasure trove of details. It may strike such a well that you won't need to even ask structured follow-up questions.

What was your dream about?

The intent of this question is to have your

child share more details about their dream. To further customize it and have them recognize that you have listened intently to them up to this point, you could frame it using their response to your initial question. For example, if they answered that their dream was boring, you could say something like, "What happened in your dream that had you experience it as boring?"

How did the dream make you feel?
Asking this can help you to know your child even better on an emotional level, keying you into feelings that they are working through. This may provide you with direct access to a situation that you weren't aware your child was facing and how they felt about it. Or it may help you to further clarify how your little one feels about a challenge or an opportunity about which you know. By asking about what was emotionally kindled for them owing to the dream, it can help them to feel more confident that you are interested in their feelings. Another benefit is that it helps them develop language skills to express their emotions.

Did the dream (or something specific in the dream) remind you of something in your life?
This can help you, and them, understand what may have inspired the dream. It can reflect what may be top of mind for your child in their life. This question also creates an opportunity for them to share a concern they have or an achievement they've

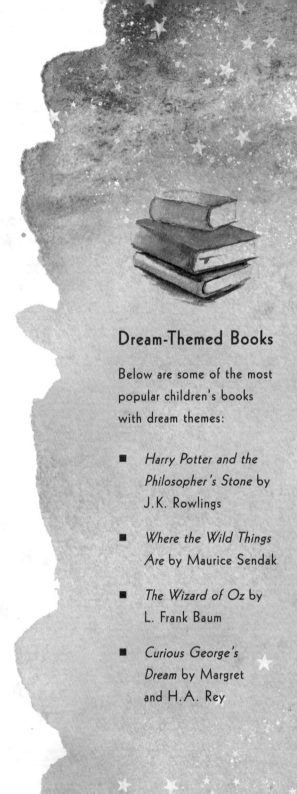

Dream-Themed Books

Below are some of the most popular children's books with dream themes:

- *Harry Potter and the Philosopher's Stone* by J.K. Rowlings

- *Where the Wild Things Are* by Maurice Sendak

- *The Wizard of Oz* by L. Frank Baum

- *Curious George's Dream* by Margret and H.A. Rey

experienced about which you may not have known. By discussing this, and seeing the dream through this lens, you may help them to understand how they may be able to further process what they are experiencing in their waking life.

What did the dream teach you?

Your child may be able to immediately perceive some important lessons that the dream gifted them. Or it may be through the recounting of the dream, and the discussions that you have, that they will discover important lessons and further understanding about themselves. As dreams can provide problem-solving awareness, explore with your child what they learned from the dream. This could run the gamut and may include relationship skills, ways to navigate a current challenge at school, and even an idea that helps them to realize how to approach a demanding homework assignment.

What is something new you're thinking about after having the dream?

This is a follow-up line of inquiry you could use to help further bridge the dream to their waking life, supporting them to take what they learned and integrate it. It will have them connect to a declaration of intent and awareness, galvanizing their confidence that they feel more skilled and adept.

WORKING THE DREAM

Since dreams are unique to the dreamer and you want your little ones to feel a sense of agency toward them, it's important when reflecting on their dream to always start by saying, "If this were my dream..." This avoids it appearing that what you think of their dream is the absolute reality, leaving no space for them to find meanings that are more personal to them.

If your child had a striking dream, whether inspiring or upsetting, encourage them to express it with artwork. They can take a dream image or scene and paint or draw it. Or perhaps sculpting it with clay or playdough is more up their alley. Alternatively, the scene in their dream may be one that is perfect to be acted out in a play. It can even serve as an idea for a mini-theater production that they can do with their friends or siblings. Or let's say that in their dream, they were exploring a new skill and they found it challenging; you can then set aside time to do that activity together, imparting to them insights and firsthand experience.

MAINTAIN AN ENCOURAGING STANCE

Sharing dreams provides you with another opportunity to praise your child. Laud them about something related to their dream. It could be its creative quality, an act of bravery they took in the dream, how much they remember about their dream, or the like. When asking your child about their dream, make sure to hold space for them in an open and nonjudgmental manner. Be conscientious about any bias you may have, whether about the process of dreaming itself or something that may arise in their dreams. Remember that what they share with you may be outside of your comfort zone or your sense of usual; for example, you may be astounded by your little one's dream recall and the amount of details that they remember. And while this may initially shock you, be careful how you respond so that they don't feel that there's anything out of the ordinary about it.

Make sure to validate their feelings. For example, if your child spoke about a dream that frightened them, you could note something like, "I understand how you may have felt scared." In this case, you could also tell them how you have scary dreams on occasion as well, so that they know that you share another commonality. Or if they recall something that perplexed them in the dream, even if it's something that seems to have an obvious meaning to you, saying something like "I understand how you may have been confused" can go a long way to making them feel seen and heard.

Throughout the process, it's good to incorporate the language that they used to mirror back when you ask them questions or make declarative statements. This will help them feel validated. Remember that a child will share their dreams in an age-appropriate way. You may even find that if a dream was significant to them and they retell it later in their life, the way that they share it will change.

MAKE DREAM SHARING A ROUTINE

Make talking about dreams a routine part of your family dynamic. Choose a time at which you ask about their dream. Perhaps it's when they first wake up, or when you're sitting down to breakfast. On the days you forget, don't be surprised if very dream-curious kids bring up the subject. If your child gets the dream bug, they may even start asking family members about them at holiday gatherings. And, as we explored in chapter 12, regularly sharing dreams helps people better remember them. Therefore, by encouraging this as a regular conversation, your kids — and you — will better recall your oneiric visions.

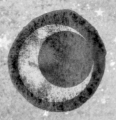

Jung and Youngsters' Dreams

As discussed in the Introduction, Carl Jung was a pioneer of depth psychology who is revered, along with Sigmund Freud, for his role in recatalyzing society's attention toward the revelatory power of dreams. Viewing children's dreams through a Jungian perspective, we can see that some may provide a child with greater self-awareness, while others may help the child anticipate future events. And while Jung noted that many children's dreams may relate to everyday life events, he also said that they were capable of having what he called big dreams, the ones that are revelatory and contain mythic archetypes. A recent addition to his available work, the 2010 publishing of *Children's Dreams*, features four years' worth of seminar presentations Jung gave on this topic.

Of course, you don't want to pressure your children to talk about their dreams. It's important to respect their privacy and how they want to honor this part of their lives. If your child doesn't seem interested in discussing their dreams, and you still want to keep the subject alive, you can note on occasion something about the dream you had, even if it's just something neutral like "I had such an interesting dream last night." This still allows for there to be an understanding that dreams are something that are normal — things that people have, talk about, and share.

KEEPING A DREAM JOURNAL

Encourage your children to document their dreams. Have them keep a dream journal that they can write in whenever they want. For kids who are starting to learn to write, this can be another great way for them to develop this skill. If your child isn't old enough to write, ask them if they want you to write it down for them. Since drawing is not only an accessible way to express the visual language of dreams but is something that most kids like to do, make sure that the journal has some blank pages. They can use these to draw, color, finger-paint, or doodle images from their dreams, or visually represent the tone of the dream, or how it made them feel.

Some children like to keep a diary. You can ask them if they want to include their dreams there or in a separate book. Remind them that since their dream journal, like their dreams, is very special, they should designate a cherished spot in which to keep it. Depending upon your child and their age, keeping their journal private, and only accessed by others by invitation, may be important.

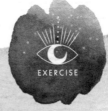

EXERCISE

Designing Their Dream Journal

To further forge your child's connection with their dream journal, have them design it themselves. To do so:

- Let them choose a notebook that they would like to use for their journal.

- Ask them what they want to call their journal and then have them write it on the cover (if they are too young, you can write it for them).

- Provide them with markers, paint, rubber stamps, and even glitter so that they can create a unique dream journal cover.

Nightmares and Night Terrors

It may be very upsetting to watch your children deal with the fear inspired by scary dreams. Know, though, that episodic nightmares are not abnormal, and in fact are more commonplace in children than in adults. They happen for kids of all ages and across genders, although there are some differences: throughout childhood, girls and boys have been found to have nightmares at similar rates until they become teenagers, a period when girls report having them more frequently than boys.

As they begin to develop their wayfinding in the world, children are faced with a multitude of firsts to experience and unknowns to navigate. Additionally, they may feel less in control than adults while connecting to age-appropriate fears. Some of these concerns may find a way to pepper their dreams, ideally so that they can give voice to them, work them out, and grow past them. However, these dream visions may, of course, be quite disconcerting.

Know that not every bad dream is a nightmare. Some children may report a dream as being scary but not find themselves emotionally disturbed as they may be from a nightmare. Generally, nightmares are those that are so vivid and emotionally inciting that they shake us up out of sleep. Note that while episodic nightmares may be normal, if your child has them very frequently or experiences ones that are so terrifying that they cause them undue anxiety or a fear of sleeping, getting professional help may be of benefit. Especially if your child has nightmares, you may want to make sure that they feel as safe as possible when they go to bed. Many of the relaxation rituals and bedroom-designing tips in the previous chapter can help with this. Remind them that they can always talk to you about what happens in their dreams and that doing so may even help their nightmares to subside.

If your child has a nightmare, don't dismiss their fear, while still strongly taking a position of offering them reassurance. And even if it seems like a means of providing them with solace, be cautious not to discount their dreams. Be careful not to say, "It was only a dream," as this will send a mixed message to them about the veracity and import of their dreams. Rather, in this instance, encourage them to remember that dreams may seem very realistic when we are sleeping, but that we always wake up from them, and that they cannot harm us.

Hearing about your child's nightmares may be like a bull's-eye arrow that gives you immediate access into understanding the roots of their upset and consternation. Based upon this, look to see what may be triggering them in their daily life and see if resolution can be made. Remember, too, that as your child works through the issues with which they may be struggling, not only will things in their waking life resolve, but their dreams will, as well. And their nightmares may abate.

As discussed in chapter 7, the phenomenon of night terrors is different than nightmares. Night terrors are experienced much more frequently by children than adults, with kids ages four to eight having them in the greatest concentration. The good news is that they are something that most kids outgrow by twelve years of age.

IMAGE REHEARSAL THERAPY

There are numerous ways that you can help comfort a child who has a nightmare. While chapter 8 addresses nightmares in general, there may be some information in there that you may find beneficial for your child. One of the concepts discussed there is Image Rehearsal Therapy (IRT), an adaptation of which has been found to be helpful for children. If your child's nightmares are rather tenacious, consider consulting with a health-care practitioner who can provide them with a systematic approach to this treatment. However, if their nightmares are less frequent or intense, you may want to see if you can use some of its principles, helping your child directly. As you are tucking your child in and talking with them about their dreams, you can discover if they previously had one that was upsetting to them. If so, ask them if they want to talk about it more.

First, help normalize their nightmares. Have them realize that most kids have them, and that there is nothing strange about them. Confidently tell them that there are things that you can do together to help the nightmares dissipate. Remind them that these dreams are not an attribute of who they are — like their physical appearance or personality — but rather something that they do, and so there are things that they can undertake to have them disappear.

Next, tell them you know a game (or strategy, if that's more age-appropriate) that helps many people fend off nightmares. Then ask them if they want to take a bad dream that they just had and come up with a better ending or resolution for it. This may be very empowering for them, as it helps them directly face their fears and exercise their creative control.

Common Themes of Children's Nightmares

- An animal trying to eat them
- Being chased
- Drowning
- Tidal waves
- Losing something
- Bugs
- Monsters
- Being alone
- Falling down

Listen in as they rescript the story line of their dream, providing prompts and encouragement where you see fit. Ask them how they feel about this new dream. Then ask if they would want to have this alternative-ending dream. If they say yes, have them concentrate in their mind's eye upon this revised dream before going to sleep. Tell them that with this exercise, there's a good chance that they may have this new dream, but if they don't, not to worry, as sometimes it takes a little extra time and work for new things to take hold. Chances are, though, that after doing this exercise several times, they may not have their bad dream again. (This exercise is an adaption of Image Rehearsal Therapy, which we explored in chapter 8.)

You could also do this rescripting exercise during the daytime and use it as a foundation for their artwork. Have them not only create a new ending for the dream in words, but also as a drawing, painting, dance, or other form of creative expression that interests them. Given that dreams are so visual, this may help them to further tap into a way to sculpt this reimagining.

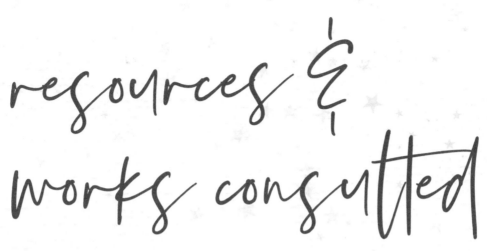

resources & works consulted

Want to learn more about sleep and dreams? Here are some of my favorite books, including those that forged the foundations of *The Complete Book of Dreams*.

Sleep

- *At Day's Close: Nights in Times Past* by A. Roger Ekirch
- *Sleep and Wakefulness* by Nathaniel Kleitman
- *The Promise of Sleep* by William C. Dement
- *The Secret Life of Sleep* by Kat Duff
- *The Sleep Revolution: Transforming Your Life, One Night at a Time* by Arianna Huffington
- *Why We Sleep: Unlocking the Power of Sleep and Dreams* by Matthew Walker

Dreams

- *Asclepius: Collection and Interpretation of Testimonies* by Emma and Ludwig Edelstein
- *Dreaming: A Very Short Introduction* by J. Allan Hobson
- *Dreaming in the World's Religions: A Comparative History* by Kelly Bulkeley
- *Dreaming the Divine* by Scott Cunningham
- *Dreams* by Carl G. Jung
- *Dreams, a Portal to the Source* by Edward C. Whitmont and Sylvia Brinton Perera
- *Dreams: Visions of the Night* by David Coxhead and Susan Hiller
- *Dreamtime and Dreamwork: Decoding the Language of the Night* edited by Stanley Krippner
- *Healing Dream and Ritual* by C. A. Meier

- *Healing Night: The Science and Spirit of Sleeping, Dreaming, and Awakening* by Rubin Naiman
- *Inner Work: Using Dreams and Active Imagination for Personal Growth* by Robert A. Johnson
- *Living Your Dreams* by Gayle M. Delaney
- *Our Dreaming Mind* by Robert L. Van de Castle
- *The Art of Dreaming* by Jill Mellick
- *The Committee of Sleep* by Deidre Barrett
- *The Dream and the Underworld* by James Hillman
- *The Healing Power of Dreams* by Patricia Garfield
- *The Interpretation of Dreams* by Sigmund Freud
- *The Practice of Dream Healing* by Edward Tick
- *The Secret History of Dreaming* by Robert Moss
- *The Tibetan Art of Dream Analysis* by Nida Chenagtsang
- *Turning Nightmares into Dreams* by Barry Krakow
- *Understanding Your Child's Dreams* by Pam Spurr
- *Why We Dream: The Transformative Power of Our Nightly Journey* by Alice Robb
- *Working with Dreams* by Montague Ullman and Nan Zimmerman
- *Writers Dreaming: 26 Writers Talk About Their Dreams and the Creative Process* by Naomi Epel

Lucid Dreaming

- *Dream Yoga* by Andrew Holecek
- *Dreams: How to Connect with Your Dreams to Enrich Your Life* by Tree Carr
- *Exploring the World of Lucid Dreaming* by Stephen LaBerge and Howard Rheingold
- *Learn to Lucid Dream* by Kristen LaMarca

Children's Dreams

- *Children's Dreams* by Kelly Bulkeley and Patricia M. Bulkley
- *Children's Dreams: Notes from the Seminar Given in 1936–1940* by Carl G. Jung

- *The Dream Book: A Young Person's Guide to Understanding Dreams* by Patricia Garfield
- *Understanding Your Child's Dreams* by Pam Spurr

Dream Symbols

- *Dictionary of Symbols* by Jean Chevalier and Alain Gheerbrant
- *Oneirocritica* by Artemidorus
- *The Book of Symbols* by Archive for Research in Archetypal Symbolism

Astrology, Tarot, and I Ching

- *Essence of the Tarot: Modern Reflections on Ancient Wisdom* by Megan Skinner
- *Planetary Apothecary* by Stephanie Gailing
- *Planets in Play* by Laurence Hillman
- *The Book of Astronomy by Guido Bonatti* translated by Benjamin N. Dykes
- *The I Ching, or, Book of Changes* translated by Richard Wilhelm and Cary F. Baynes
- *The Rulership Book* by Rex E. Bills
- *You Were Born for This: Astrology for Radical Self-Acceptance* by Chani Nicholas

Healing Remedies

- *Aromatherapy for Healing the Spirit* by Gabriel Mojay
- *Dreams, Symbols & Homeopathy* by Jane Cicchetti
- *Flower Essence Repertory* by Patricia Kaminski and Richard Katz
- *Flower Power* by Anne McIntyre
- *The Complete German Commission E Monographs* by Mark Blumenthal et al.
- *The Crystal Bible* by Judy Hall
- *The Encyclopedia of Bach Flower Therapy* by Mechthild Scheffer
- *The Phoenix Repertory* by Dr. JPS Bakshi

For Astrology Information

- Find calendars for New Moons, as well as Mercury, Venus, and Mars Retrograde, at stephaniegailing.com
- Find your Sun, Moon, and Ascendant sign at astro.com or sodivine.us

acknowledgments

The Complete Book of Dreams is a dream come true for me, one made possible by a stellar array of people who have supported and inspired me, and to whom I am eternally grateful:

John Foster, editor extraordinaire, whose vision shaped this book from its inception, and whose confidence in me as a writer is a gift that I will always treasure. The amazing team at Wellfleet — including Publisher Rage Kindelsperger, Creative Director Laura Drew, Managing Editor Cara Donaldson, and Marketing Manager Lydia Anderson — for creating this beautiful book and sharing it with the world. And to Sosha Davis for her gorgeous artwork and Designer Kate Smith for her impeccable graphic design.

My husband Sebastiano and stepdaughter Simone, who light up my heart every day. My mother Bernice, who not only remembers her dreams more extensively than anyone I know, but whose unconditional love has allowed me to live the life of my dreams. And to the rest of my family: while I may not live near you, you are closer to me than you even know.

Aimee Hartstein and Heidi Lender, for being the best friends a girl could ever hope for. Laurence Hillman, my inspiring mentor and friend. Sherene Schostak, Megan Skinner, Tony Howard, and Tali Edut, my colleagues who are more like family, and who helped me give voice to my ideas over the years.

All the philosophers, artists, scientists, health-care professionals, and laypersons who have been fascinated by their dreams, and whose curiosity and passion have helped us to better understand our own. And you, dear reader: may your dreams inspire you to live your dream life and help others to do the same.

about the author

Stephanie Gailing is a life guide, modern mystic, and author with more than twenty-five years of experience. Her unique approach to healing weaves together compassion-based coaching, wellness strategies, dreamwork, and astrological insights. In addition to working directly with individuals, couples, and organizations throughout the world, Stephanie regularly teaches workshops and writes about holistic well-being, inspiring her audience with ways to live their dream life. Co-host of the *So Divine!* podcast, Stephanie is also the author of *Planetary Apothecary*, a pioneering book in the field of wellness astrology. She holds a Certificate in EcoPsychology from Pacifica University, an Advanced Diploma in Coaching from New York University, and an MS in Nutrition from Bastyr University. Stephanie lives in Seattle with her husband Sebastiano. You can find more about her and her work at StephanieGailing.com.

index